Everyone Has a Tipped Uterus:

69 Things Your Gynecologist Wishes You Knew

D1715975

Melissa Wolf, MD

First published by Dog Ear Publishing
4010 W. 86th Street, Ste H
Indianapolis, IN 46268
www.dogearpublishing.net

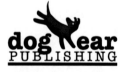

ISBN: 978-1-4575-1003-8

This book is printed on acid-free paper.

Printed in the United States of America

For my patients

Introduction

The inspiration for this book came from a trip to the auto mechanic. I know nothing about cars but had a persistent emergency light on, a grinding sound coming from the brakes, and a strong sensation that the vehicle was pulling left. I took the car in, and apparently, the light was off and the other problems could not be reproduced. They charged me $200 and told me everything was fine. I felt stupid for even being there. Of course, driving home, the emergency light came back on, the brakes still made the same sound, and the vehicle still pulled left. It was frustrating to know that everything had allegedly been evaluated thoroughly and deemed fine yet I still noticed the same problems. Clearly, I hadn't communicated my car symptoms correctly. As I don't know how the car works, or what is normal versus not, I did not feel reassured when I left with the same problems I had gone in with.

As a gynecologist (women's health doctor), this experience prompted me to consider how patients in my office must feel. Women present with concerns that I often feel are normal and nothing to worry about. I sometimes am nonchalant about dismissing their concerns as normal and moving on. It occurred to me that just as I am worried that the grinding sound of the brakes means that I might crash and die at anytime from brake failure, a patient might be worried that mid-cycle menstrual spotting means she has uterine cancer. Of course, my brakes are fine, and mid-cycle spotting is a common occurrence with normal ovulation; however, our fears are similar.

This book is designed to address some of the most common things that I believe worry patients and to give tips on how to best navigate a gynecologic appointment. If I had gone to the auto mechanic with a friend knowledgeable about cars who could ask the right questions and describe my problems using the right lingo, I might have felt more confident about the final vehicle diagnosis. This book is your insider guide to the gynecology office, including how to handle the potentially embarrassing situation of seeing your gynecologist in public! The information described here is intended to enhance your knowledge of certain aspects of women's health and should not replace the advice of your personal physician. Please speak directly with your doctor if you have any health concerns.

Contents

1.

Is There an Egg in Your Vagina?

I must admit, I chuckled when a woman called to report she had a cell phone stuck in her vagina and wondered what to do; however, only for a moment. As gynecologists, we have heard everything. Believe it or not, we already know about your most embarrassing and awkward situations. We have removed tampons forgotten in the vagina for weeks. We know of vaginal sex, oral sex, anal sex, sex toys, sex parties, and casual sex. We assume monogamy is the exception, not the norm. We won't bat an eye if you request chlamydia testing and have been married for 20 years. We have stitched vaginal lacerations in the emergency room at 3 a.m. from toys that didn't fit or partners who were too vigorous. We have removed any number of objects "stuck up there," including rings, condoms, crayons, and hard-boiled eggs.

We have literally heard everything, so feel free to speak openly. If you have a question, situation, or sexual practice to discuss, let us know. Getting the facts and getting the proper infection screening is critical to your health. I completely understand that saying the words "I have an egg stuck in my vagina," or "I think I lost a tampon," is awkward; however, the solution is actually very simple. A quick office visit and you are good to go! We won't post your exam findings on Facebook or announce your predicament over the office intercom system. These situations are actually very common, and we are happy to help. No judgment. Really.

2.

What Exactly is an OBGYN?

OBGYN stands for obstetrician/gynecologist. This type of doctor has completed college, medical school, and at least four years of specialized training in delivering babies (vaginal or cesarean section), gynecologic surgery (hysterectomy, tubal ligation, laparoscopy, etc.), and women's health. He or she has limited training in general medicine. In comparison, family practitioners and internists have completed college, medical school, and at least three years of training in general medicine. Some family practitioners also have training in pregnancy and deliveries.

Many gynecologists feel they are specialists in women's health, not general practitioners. This is important to understand, because many women come to their annual exam and pap smear with a long list of medical complaints such as back pain, headaches, swollen feet, heart palpitations, hair loss, skin rashes, and joint pain. We might be able to point you in the right direction or make a referral to a general practitioner for these concerns, but we are not specifically trained to evaluate and treat conditions outside of pregnancy and gynecology.

Obstetrician/gynecologists specialize in pregnancy, breast diseases, and conditions of the ovaries, uterus, tubes, cervix, vagina, and vulva, just as a nephrologist is a specialist in kidney disease. Each gynecologist has a different level of comfort evaluating and treating conditions and symptoms outside of obstetrics and gynecology. Many women assume gynecologists will treat all their conditions and then feel the doctor has wasted her time when only a pap smear is done. The easiest way to get around this is to simply ask when you make an appointment if the doctor will address your non-gynecologic concerns. Assuming your gynecologist will treat heart palpitations is like assuming your cardiologist (heart specialist) will do a pap smear or treat your yeast infection. Also, if you need medications refilled for non-female problems like high blood pressure, high cholesterol, back pain, or ADD, ask prior to scheduling the appointment if this is something your provider is willing to do.

3.

Doctors and Hair Stylists

In medicine, as with hair stylists, accountants, babysitters, and auto mechanics, you sometimes have to meet with several different service providers before you find one you love. Don't be afraid to seek a second or third opinion for your health condition, especially if you do not trust or connect with your original provider. Even within the same field, medical doctors have many different personalities and specific areas of expertise. Likewise, naturopathic doctors, acupuncturists, and chiropractors may all offer different solutions to any given problem.

Often patients are shy about seeking different opinions or reluctant to confess that they have chosen to work with someone else. Admittedly, this discussion can feel like a bad break-up! Remember this: your doctor wants you to be happy and to connect with the personality and treatment plan you feel most comfortable with. Ultimately, we want for you what you want for yourself: to feel better. Most providers view themselves as health consultants, not the final solution to every problem. You, as a patient, are consulting a physician for a health condition to see if we can explain why you are experiencing certain symptoms and to see if we have any strategies to help you feel better. If your doctor proposes a solution that you are comfortable with, fantastic; if not, feel free to shop around.

Also, just because you have had one or 100 appointments in any office or with any single physician does not mean you cannot change. Offices will happily supply medical records, send letters, or speak with your new provider, whoever that may be. You do not have to hide from your former doctor in the supermarket or worry that we are upset with you. We understand that you are searching for a solution that we may not have or that our personalities may not mesh. However, don't hesitate to return for a consult if you have been away for awhile. Most physicians will gladly welcome the opportunity to reconnect with former patients and are very unlikely to quiz you as to why you sought advice elsewhere. Most commonly we will be curious as to whether you found a solution to your original problem and may ask you to describe what ultimately helped you so we can share this success strategy with others.

4.

I Won't Remember Your Vagina

My nurse is constantly amazed at how little I remember. She will ask me about a patient I saw earlier in the week and I will have literally no recollection of the visit without looking at the chart and reviewing my notes. She will try to give me prompts such as "the lady who works at the lumber yard and has six kids and was here with a rash and had her spleen removed and had the skeleton tattoo"…honestly, no recollection. I promise, I won't remember doing your pap smear if I see you outside the office. This is true for most physicians, although some are better than others about remembering names and personal information.

Over the years, many women have told me they are mortified when they see me in public because I did their pap smear or genital exam. For perspective, I sometimes do 15 or more female exams in a single day. All day, I look at lesions, bumps, warts, and normal anatomy. Some women shave or wax, some don't. Some have piercings, some don't. If you see me in Wal-Mart, I may not remember meeting you at all, let alone what your female parts looked like or what piercings you had. Honestly, I am usually the one horrified at my personal inability to remember patients I have met in my office.

Also, outside the hospital, I am often wearing casual sweatpants covered in dog fur or running tights, and feel personally distressed about my nonprofessional appearance when I unexpectedly encounter one of my patients. One of my most embarrassing moments was when a pregnant patient spotted me crawling around on the floor in PetSmart trying to coax my German shepherd, Maya, to participate in puppy class instead of hiding behind the cat litter. The patient approached me looking confused and asked hesitantly, "Are you my doctor?" just as Maya peed on the floor and made a break for the door knocking down a store display shelf as she ran. Perfect. Who do you think was more embarrassed?

The best course of action if you see your doctor outside the office is to smile, wave, ask them about the weather, or ignore them completely, but don't worry for even a second that your doctor might be snickering to him- or herself about your gynecologic appointment, sexual practices, or physical exam.

5.

Doctors Can Smell Marijuana

Even though we spent most of college in the library, doctors are familiar with the scent of marijuana. I know, you quit last year; however, we can still smell it. Several of my patients reek so strongly of marijuana that I feel woozy just being in the room with them. Some of these same patients report they don't smoke. The same is true for tobacco. I recently cared for a pregnant patient with high blood pressure who smoked two packs a day and claimed she had quit, yet at every appointment, her breath and clothes smelled so strongly of tobacco that I felt like I had smoked a pack of Marlboros myself after being in her presence. Alcohol is no different. If you are drunk at your appointment, we can tell.

The bottom line is, your doctor has no intention of judging your social habits. Your doctor does, however, need to know the truth about what you are using so as not to prescribe a medication that could interact dangerously with any given substance. The doctor also needs to be able to advise you of potential health risks linked to certain practices and to offer treatment. If you decline to get treatment for substance use, that is absolutely your decision, but lying about it is not a great strategy, especially when you reek of a given chemical.

Incidentally, your doctor was likely taught in medical school to double whatever amount of any given substance you admit to using. For example: If you state, "I smoke marijuana once a week," we are taught to assume that you smoke marijuana at least twice a week (double what you reported). Asking questions about substance use is not designed to upset, offend, or criticize you. These questions are part of a basic health assessment. In my own life, I watched one of my relatives attend numerous doctor visits and report drinking one glass of wine per night when the truth was actually one *bottle* of bourbon per night. No physician ever pressed her, and she didn't end up receiving treatment for her underlying depression or getting help with alcohol addiction until she was in her mid 50s. Understandably, you might feel hesitant to discuss these topics; however, your doctor can generally be much more helpful if you provide accurate and truthful information. After all, are you paying your physician to conceal your habits or to help you improve your health?

6.

Have STD Testing (Especially for Chlamydia) with Each New Sexual Partner

Chlamydia and other sexually transmitted infections are generally asymptomatic in men. Also, men are much less likely to go to a doctor if they have a symptom, and many men have no idea that they are infected with chlamydia, herpes, HPV, HIV, etc. Every time you have a new sexual partner, you should assume that you have been infected with something. This is especially true if you do not use condoms. Yes, I know, you always use condoms (except when you were camping, or when you drank too much, or when you were on vacation, or when he forgot to wear one)! Chlamydia can climb up through the cervix, through the uterus, and into the fallopian tubes, causing scarring and subsequent infertility. This means that if you have chlamydia and you don't know it, you might not be able to get pregnant in the future. The test is easy, the treatment is easy, and you have no excuse not to get tested…with each new partner.

Chlamydia testing is currently recommended for sexually active women through the age of 26 at least once a year; however, if you are 17 and had three partners in one year, this means you should have three chlamydia tests that year (no, we won't tell your mother). The same goes for other sexually transmitted infections. Don't worry that your gynecologist will be upset with you or be shocked that you had ten sexual partners (or 100 partners) in one year. We have heard everything and really do not care what your personal sexual practices are. We only want to prevent you from transmitting disease to others and from being harmed yourself.

Regarding confidentiality, your doctor cannot and will not tell your spouse, your mother, your sister, your employer, or anyone else about your office visit or test results without your permission. If, however, you do not have your own health insurance and are a member on another person's policy (teenagers and wives, beware), consider that the policy holder may receive notification of your visit in the form of a bill from the insurance company. This can lead to uncomfortable conversations if you are not prepared. If you are concerned about incidental disclosure via insurance billing, consider going to a free clinic for your testing, or pay out of pocket (don't bill the insurance) at your usual doctor's office. Brainstorm creative payment plans, but don't avoid or delay getting tested for confidentiality or insurance concerns.

7.

Everyone Has a Tipped Uterus

Did you know, *every* woman's uterus is tipped? At least once a day, usually during a pap smear, I hear from patients that a prior doctor told them their uterus was "tipped" or "tilted" and they have been worrying about it ever since. Also, oddly enough, when I look at what drives Internet traffic to my pregnancy website, FlutterFacts.com, I find that a Google search for "tipped uterus" is the hands down winner. This seems to distress many women, and yet it is not only common, but totally normal. FYI, you can become pregnant even with a "tipped" uterus.

A normal position for a uterus is tipped forward (anteverted), tipped backward (retroverted), straight (midposition), or deviated (tilted) to the right or left. The uterus is not glued in one spot inside the pelvis. It moves around your low belly the way your tongue moves inside your mouth. While you can control how your tongue moves, you cannot move your own uterus voluntarily. The uterus is attached to the upper vagina by the cervix and to the pelvic sidewalls by ligaments, but it moves up, down, right, and left all the time. The position of the uterus means nothing. Let me say it again: the position of the uterus means *nothing*. It is only relevant in special circumstances such as during the placement of an IUD (intrauterine device). In this case, your doctor needs to know the exact trajectory of your uterus to position the IUD properly. If the uterine position cannot be felt during a physical exam, an ultrasound can be used to clarify.

Sometimes a woman with a sharply retroverted uterus that is tipped backward at an acute angle can have pain with intercourse because during sex, the penis hits the top of the uterus. Also, these women might have more intestinal symptoms like diarrhea, or urgency to move their bowels during their men-strual periods because the backward tipped uterus can press on the rectum. These symptoms can be very annoying, but they are not dangerous. It is usually very easy to tell on a pelvic exam which way the uterus is tipped, so, if you want to know, ask your doctor during your gynecologic exam.

8.

Your Ovaries Are Not in Your Mid-abdomen

"My ovary hurts," is one of the most commonly reported concerns in my office. More often than not, a patient reports this and then points to a place on her mid-abdomen near the belly button to indicate the location of her pain. Unfortunately, this is not where the ovaries are located anatomically. It can be very challenging for me to convince a woman pointing to her belly button that it is not her ovaries causing pain in that area. I know, in grade school and all over the Internet, that diagram of the uterus with the tubes/ovaries projecting out like antlers to each side prevails; however, in reality, this is not how these organs are positioned inside your body. For most women, the ovaries are located *behind* the uterus, near the top of the vagina. It is nearly impossible to point to your ovaries through your belly.

To palpate (feel) an ovary during a physical exam, your doctor has to push down really hard on your lower belly to feel it internally with the vaginal hand. If you have pain, I'm not suggesting that your ovary doesn't hurt; however, I am suggesting that it is probably not your ovary causing discomfort if the pain is in your mid-abdomen. In fact, most of the time, abdominal pain in women is related to the intestine or digestive tract, especially if the discomfort is located in the mid or upper belly. By taking a medical history and completing a physical exam, your doctor can help you discover what exactly is causing your pain. I encourage you to be open to the idea that something other than your ovary may be the source.

9.

Ovarian Cysts Are Normal

Yikes! Really? Yes. Believe it or not, most ovarian cysts are normal. Did you know that *every month* from puberty to menopause, your ovary produces an egg, and as part of this normal process of egg production, an ovarian cyst forms? After the egg pops out of the ovary (ovulation), if you are not pregnant, the cyst goes away, and a few weeks later, the cycle starts again. If you are pregnant, the cyst and surrounding tissue produce progesterone to help keep the pregnancy alive. The cyst then usually goes away in early pregnancy. A cyst can often be seen on normal ovaries for at least two out of the four weeks of a normal menstrual cycle and sometimes longer. This means that if you have a pelvic ultrasound to "check your ovaries" a cyst will often be present.

"How do I know if my ovarian cyst is normal?" The key is in its size and consistency. If the cyst is less than 5 cm and is filled with clear fluid, it is usually normal. A cyst is abnormal if it is filled with blood or solid material. These characteristics can typically be seen on ultrasound. A cyst larger than 5 cm or a cyst filled with blood is often observed for 4–12 weeks to see if it will resolve on its own, as they often do. If it does not go away on its own, surgery to drain the cyst is an option. A cyst filled with solid material is often surgically removed, as these do not generally go away spontaneously. An ovarian cyst found in a menopausal woman may be followed more closely as these women should not be ovulating (producing eggs), and therefore not creating cysts after menopause.

"My cyst ruptured; what does that mean?" Women diagnosed with ruptured cysts are often very concerned about their ovaries.

They envision their ovaries exploding, malfunctioning, or becoming cancerous; however, every month since puberty, your ovaries have likely created an ovarian cyst that has subsequently ruptured (burst). This describes the normal process of ovulation. Sometimes, if the cyst is large or full of blood, both the cyst and the rupture can be painful. Even when it is painful, a ruptured cyst is usually a good thing. Why? Because it means that the cyst is in the process of going away. Ruptured means it is draining its contents (usually clear fluid or blood) into the pelvis. The fluid or blood will be naturally reabsorbed by the body, and the ovary will return to normal. This process usually takes 2–12 weeks.

"When should I have surgery for my ovarian cyst?" Surgery is almost *never* needed for an ovarian cyst, as most cysts are normal and take care of themselves. If the ovary is twisted on itself (torsed), surgery is required at that time; however, this situation is rare and women with this condition are usually *extremely* ill with pain, fever, vomiting, and other symptoms. If the ovary is not twisted, as in most cases, ultrasound follow-up is commonly recommended in 4–12 weeks to see if the cyst is gone. If the cyst has gotten larger or looks very different than before, you may be offered surgery at that time depending on your age and symptoms.

10.

A Normal Menstrual Cycle Is 21–35 Days Long

Women often report the strangest phenomenon. They state that their menstrual period *always* comes on the sixth of the month but during the present cycle, it was abnormal because it came on the third. Funny. A normal cycle is 21–35 days long and does usually recur at a similar interval for individuals. For example, if my current cycle is 26 days, my next cycle is likely to be 26 days, but keep in mind, it could be anywhere from 21 to 35 days long. Because the months of the calendar vary from 28 to 31 days, it is therefore amazing that a menstrual period would always occur on the identical monthly calendar date. Most cycles are 27–31 days or so, and this roughly approximates the monthly calendar system but could rarely be exact.

Variations in cycle length are common, so don't be alarmed if the calendar date varies from time to time, or if you have two periods in the same month (one at the beginning, and one at the end of the month). Noted deviations from the norm can be understandably worrisome for some women. To alleviate your concerns, ask yourself if your current cycle was between 21 and 35 days. If the answer is yes, then you most likely had a normal menstrual cycle. If you are bleeding more or less often, consider discussing this with your physician.

Also, remember that to calculate the length of your menstrual cycle, start counting from day 1, which is the first day of bleeding, to the subsequent cycle's day 1. The cycle length is not the number of days between the end of one period and the start of the next. It is the number of days from the *start* of one period to the start of the next cycle. It is a good idea to track your menstrual bleeding on a calendar so that if you develop a problem with your periods in the future, your doctor can see what your typical pattern is like and understand any current changes. It is common for the amount of bleeding and cycle length to change over time, after each pregnancy, or in your mid 40s as you approach menopause.

11.

The Only Way to Diagnose Endometriosis Is with Laparoscopy

Endometriosis is a common condition in women. It means that there are cells usually only found *inside* the uterus identified *outside* the uterus. Just as the cells inside the uterus bleed every month and cause a menstrual period, if these cells are outside the uterus, they can also bleed, causing irritation and pelvic pain. The exact cause of endometriosis is unknown. It is typically treated with a combination of hormone therapy such as birth control pills, surgery, and anti-inflammatory medications. Here's the catch: The only way to know for certain if you have endometriosis is with surgery. We must put a camera inside your belly and look for the endometriosis implants outside the uterus. If we see an area that appears to be endometriosis, we take a sample (biopsy) and send it to the lab for confirmation. Endometriosis cannot be seen on an ultrasound, seen on a CT scan, or determined by your pap smear.

Sometimes a description of symptoms and findings on physical exam suggest that you may have this condition, but the only way to know for sure is with surgery. Women often report that they have *severe* endometriosis as part of their medical history, yet they have never had surgery to actually confirm this condition. If and when surgery is subsequently done, there is often no endometriosis to be found. Understandably, this leads to confusion and anger about the former diagnosis as women have often lived with this medical label for years and believed it to be the source of their pain or fertility problem. It is important to remember that just because your mother had endometriosis does not mean that you automatically have this condition. Just because someone told you that you might have endometriosis based on certain symptoms does not mean that you truly do. It is best to avoid formally labeling yourself with this condition unless it has been properly diagnosed with surgical assessment and biopsy.

If you currently carry a diagnosis of "endometriosis" and have not had surgery, talk with your doctor about why he or she believes that you may have this condition. Understanding how your provider is thinking can help you understand your symptoms and the relevant treatment options. The main reason doctors do not operate on every patient suspected to have endometriosis is because the surgery itself often is not a cure, especially for mild disease. Even when we make a formal diagnosis through surgery, the treatment is usually still medical and requires using certain medications to suppress the endometriosis that you may have. Because the surgery itself is not the actual cure, many doctors prefer to use medication to improve your pain without putting you through the rigors and stress of an operation.

12.

Never Use Douche

Douche is a product sold over the counter that women spray inside the vagina to "clean themselves." It can also be homemade with vinegar or yogurt. Many women commonly use douche after intercourse, after their periods, or if they feel they have a vaginal infection. Tell your friends: Douche is *never* needed. The vaginal tissue produces mucus and discharge in much the same way the mouth produces saliva. These secretions help keep the pH and the normal vaginal bacteria in balance. If you spray vinegar or any commercial product into the vagina, this pH balance is disrupted and many of the normal bacteria are killed. This imbalance can lead to overgrowth of yeast or of infectious bacteria and can cause vaginal itching and irritation. Let your body do what it is designed to do. The "need" for douche is created by successful marketing and is not necessary…ever.

The same goes for yogurt soaked tampons. There is no reason to ever place a tampon soaked in anything (yogurt, vinegar, alcohol, iodine, etc.) inside your vagina. Yes, people really do soak tampons in vodka and insert them vaginally for various reasons. Please use tampons for their intended purpose of menstrual blood absorption only. Incidentally, if you are afraid to use tampons or are not sure how to place one correctly, ask your gynecologist about this. Even if you have never touched a tampon before in your life, we can instruct you in their proper (and painless) use within about five minutes during an office appointment.

13.

Wash Only with Water

I know this sounds outrageous. *No soap?! It's dirty down there! Yuck!* Seriously, I mean no soap. Do not apply lotions or sprays or perfumes or wipes or anything other than water to the vulva or vagina. This area is very sensitive, and most people are allergic to whatever chemicals they are applying. Wondering why you have a burning sensation or itching? Could be an infection (see your doctor immediately for testing) or, more likely, it is the new body wash you got online. Scrap the soap and see how you feel. Putting soap in your vagina is never a good idea. Period. End of story.

14.

Fumigation

Many women wear strong perfume as part of their daily routine and others apply an excessive amount prior to their gynecologic exam so they don't "smell." I promise you, the perfume is much, much, worse than your normal body odor. Showering or bathing prior to your exam is definitely preferred; however, I am begging you not to douse yourself with fragrance so you don't smell. I have done many female exams with my eyes watering, nose running, and throat swelling from an allergic reaction to fragrance someone sprayed on herself. After the exam, I can barely speak to discuss the findings and can't exit the room quickly enough. Also, sometimes, a specific vaginal odor is a critical part of the diagnosis. Bacterial vaginosis, for example, has a distinct fishy odor. If you cover it up with gardenia perfume, your provider might miss the diagnosis and you could remain untreated. I completely understand that having a gynecologic exam is uncomfortable, but if you want the best care and assessment stick with au naturale.

15.

We Don't Care if You Don't Shave Your Legs

Many women apologize profusely when they haven't shaved their legs prior to their female exam. Here's the skinny: Gynecologists are also trained in obstetrics. This means we have all delivered babies and done surgery. This also means that at some point in our lives we have been covered in amniotic fluid, blood, or worse. I personally have had amniotic fluid dripping off my chin and enough blood in my shoe to make a squishing sound when I walked. I guarantee, none of us will notice or care if you haven't shaved your legs, painted your toenails, or if your feet smell (everyone's do). No need to apologize.

16.

That Small Red Pill That Starts with the Letter D

I can't tell you the number of times patients ask me for refills on a given medication and yet do not know the name. They will state, "It is a small red pill," "It is a really low dose," or "I think it starts with the letter D," and expect me to decipher this. I strongly suggest that you come to the doctor's office, hospital, or medical clinic with a complete list of your medications. This includes the dose, the name, how many times a day or week you take the medication, and how long you have been taking it.

Asking your doctor to guess the names and doses of the medications you take is dangerous. Also, it is challenging for us to know if something we are considering prescribing might interfere with your current medications when we don't know what they are. For example, some seizure medications can be less effective when taken with birth control pills. If you don't know the name of your seizure medication, I don't know if birth control pills are a good contraceptive option for you.

Incidentally, birth control pills are considered medication; so is a Mirena IUD. A typical conversation in my office goes like this: "Are you taking any medications?" I ask.

"No."

"What about birth control pills?"

"Yes, I take those."

"What kind do you take?"

"The ones in the green package, a really low dose; I'm not sure of the name, though." (There are about 50 different types of birth control pills that could be considered low dose).

"Do you take any vitamins?"

"No."

"What about fish oil?"

"Yes, I take that."

"Anything over-the-counter?"

"No."

"What about Tylenol, Sudafed, or migraine medications?"

"I take Excedrin Migraine three times a week and Claritin for seasonal allergies."

In this example, birth control pills, fish oil, Excedrin Migraine, and Claritin would all be considered medications and should be routinely disclosed.

Remember, knowing your medications applies to all "drugs" you put into your body, including vitamins, minerals, supplements, herbal remedies, weight-loss products, potions, tinctures, medical foods, energy drinks, over-the-counter tablets—everything. All these substances interact with each other and affect your health. If you report that you are only taking birth control pills but yet you are also taking Excedrin Migraine daily, taking St John's Wort daily, drinking eight cups of weight-loss tea daily, and taking Colon Cleanse off the Internet, I am clearly missing the big picture.

It is also important that you know why you are taking a given medication or supplement. Surprisingly, many women come to the clinic with a complete list of ten medications and herbal products yet don't know what they are for. They say, "My doctor or naturopath told me to take this," but don't understand why. Dutifully taking prescriptions because your provider advised you to do so is never a good idea. Understand why you are taking something, what the side effects are, and for how long it will be needed. Also, remember that "medical" marijuana and other drugs can interfere with your medications too.

In case you were wondering, so-called "medical" marijuana is *not* safe in pregnancy. Many of my pregnant patients feel they can continue their medical marijuana for back pain or nausea during pregnancy because they have been prescribed a Green Card by a physician. Marijuana is marijuana and can affect the baby's brain development whether or not you have an official Green Card. It is best to discontinue the use of marijuana, tobacco products, alcohol (no, one drink per week is not okay), and all other drugs during pregnancy. For more comprehensive information on pregnancy, visit www.FlutterFacts.com.

17.

Don't Assume Your Gynecologist Will Prescribe the Medication You Request

Many women use their gynecologist as a primary care physician too. This means that they are seeing a doctor specifically trained in gynecology as a family physician or internist. Family physicians and internists have extensive training in general medical conditions including migraines, heart disease, thyroid disease, musculoskeletal injuries, dizziness, heartburn, high cholesterol, high blood pressure, diabetes, anxiety, leg cramps, and nausea. Gynecologists specialize in diseases and conditions of the breast, uterus, cervix, vagina, and vulva. Many gynecologists feel comfortable also acting as family physicians, but many do not. It is best not to assume that the gynecologist you have your appointment with will be comfortable refilling your seizure or blood pressure medication. Also, don't assume your gynecologist will refill chronic back pain medications, anxiety medications, diet pills, or ADD prescriptions.

If you prefer to use your gynecologist as your primary doctor, the best strategy is to simply ask when you make the appointment if the doctor will refill or prescribe the medications you want. I have unfortunately disappointed many patients over the years who requested "that testosterone patch I saw on TV" or "the diet pills my friend uses." Although we sometimes are treated as such, doctors prefer not to be viewed as PEZ dispensers for pharmaceuticals. What you saw on TV or what your friend uses might not be right or safe for you.

18.

Not All Offices Have Drug Samples

Personally, I almost never distribute prescription medication samples. Having been married to a former pharmaceutical sales rep, I learned many behind-the-scenes strategies that drug companies use to entice doctors to prescribe their specific medications. I learned of sales bonuses for numbers of prescriptions written, training and role play sessions on how to befriend providers and office staff, and numerous other incentives for sales made. We all know the pharmaceutical industry is a sales industry and naturally it rewards its employees for performance (doctors prescribing more of a given medication) in the same way that auto companies reward their employees for selling vehicles. While I am totally in favor of fair access to needed medications, using financial incentives to modify physician prescribing practices quite frankly turns my stomach. Ugh. Once I learned of these strategies, I stopped offering drug samples to my patients and declined to meet with any pharmaceutical sales reps except for rare occasions.

Prescription drug samples and sales incentives are thankfully being phased out of many clinical practices and pharmaceutical companies; however, don't assume that if you need a certain prescription, your office or doctor will have samples available. Some people are so accustomed to free medication samples that they are appalled when they actually have to pay for a prescription. Most drugs have inexpensive generic formulations or are available on a discount plan at Wal-Mart or Costco. Even without insurance, you can often find an acceptable formulation without using samples. Of course, this is not true for every medication, and some people are allergic to certain generics. If the specific medication you require is only available through a pharmaceutical company or is outrageously expensive, we will do our best to obtain it for you. The bottom line is, if you are seeing a new doctor; don't assume the office has medication samples. If you are expecting to receive drug samples at your appointment, ask the reception-ist when you schedule the office visit so that you are not disap-pointed. If cost is an issue, feel free to discuss this openly with your provider.

19.

Medication Does Not Change Rotten Relationships

Depression is a debilitating condition, and I understand you may be clinically depressed. Most of my extended family has suffered with this ailment, and I have witnessed its effects on many of my friends, relatives, and patients. Anxiety and depression are common these days; however, understanding your situation is imperative. Many women come in reporting abusive relationships, absent boyfriends, unsupportive families, and rotten marriages. They hate their jobs; they feel bored, underappreciated, unloved, and disrespected. For many, these situations have persisted for months or years. Now they come, as a seemingly last resort, to my office and request an anti-depressant, anti-anxiety, or insomnia medication to help them feel better. Could this be the answer? Maybe; however, pills are not miracles.

Pills to treat depression can be a great starting point but they do not change your marriage or your job. Using a prescription to address a relationship problem or tolerate your boss is bound to fail. If you do not acknowledge and tackle the underlying issues, you will inevitably return to my office in a few weeks and request a higher dose or a different medication, reporting that the prescription isn't working. A better strategy is to let the medication create space for you to make needed changes in your life. The drug can help you find the motivation to get a new job or find the courage to kick your boyfriend to the curb, but it will not do these things for you. I have seen anti-depressant medication thankfully bring many people back from the brink of disaster, but don't expect it to change your life without any action towards transformation on your part.

For more information on practical strategies you can use to heal yourself of depression and "the daily blahs," visit www.RedLetterHealth.com. This condition is near and dear to my heart and it is the topic of my popular presentation "Unwind Your Mind, Live Inspired!"

20.

The Doorknob Question

Ah, the famous doorknob question. It usually sounds something like, "By the way, I have no interest in sex. Is there a pill for that?" or "Sometimes I have to put one finger inside my vagina in order to have a bowel movement. Is that normal?" Clearly, these are sensitive issues that will require time, attention, and consideration to properly address. To make the most of your appointment, list all your concerns up front (including the potentially embarrassing ones), not when your doctor's hand is on the doorknob to leave the room.

If you wait for the doorknob, I really only have three choices: (1) ask you to make another appointment to discuss the issue, making you feel brushed off; (2) Discuss your concern quickly and incompletely, making you feel brushed off; or (3) Sit down, give you proper time and attention, and make the remaining patients feel brushed off because now I am an hour behind. I understand certain topics are embarrassing and difficult, but I encourage you to muster the courage to mention them early, and give your provider the opportunity to address all your concerns.

If you find yourself meeting with a doctor who seems to have his or her hand on the doorknob to leave from the moment he or she initially walks into the room to meet with you, this can be frustrating. Consider bringing a list of questions to your appointment and asking the physician to go over the list with you. If the doctor seems rushed, you could also ask him if he would like you to schedule a separate appointment to sit down and review your questions. Asking this question is a way to convey to the physician that you feel rushed and have not had your concerns addressed. In this scenario, some doctors will then sit down and spend time with you straight away, whereas others might take you up on your offer for a separate appointment. Ultimately, consider changing doctors if you feel rushed at every appointment, and especially if you feel that your concerns and questions aren't being adequately addressed.

21.

Be Brief with the Nurse and Complete with the Physician

I remember going to the pediatric office with my mom as a kid for an ear infection and listening to her describe the details of my condition in great length over and over. I always wondered why she had to repeat herself, and it wasn't until I became a physician that I realized this is the norm. Here is a hot tip: Don't repeat yourself. Tell your detailed story once, to the physician. The purpose of the receptionist is to determine how much time you will need with the physician for a given problem. The purpose of the nurse or medical assistant is to clarify your history, obtain vital signs including your weight and blood pressure, prepare the room and supplies, and provide other relevant information such as lab results and old records to the physician for your evaluation. The purpose of the physician is to evaluate your complaint and propose treatment strategies.

It is not necessary to give every detail of your story to the receptionist when you check in or to the person who is taking your blood pressure. If you have irregular menstrual cycles, state, "I have irregular periods." You do not need to review your entire menstrual calendar with all the ancillary staff prior to meeting with the physician. The best use of your time is to be brief with the receptionist and nurse and detailed with the physician. This strategy will save you time and will also allow you to be heard. You can skip wondering if the nurse told the doctor what you said and feeling annoyed that you have to repeat yourself.

22.

The Nurse Needs to Know

While I just recommended being brief with the nurse and complete with the physician in the prior section, there is such a thing as being *too* brief. The nurse does, in fact, need to know some information as to why you are in the office so she can prepare the exam room for the physician to do the correct type of evaluation. I understand it can be humiliating to visit the gynecology office. Everyone in the waiting room assumes you have chlamydia or a sexual problem—otherwise, why would you be there, right? Of course you also have to tell the receptionist why you are requesting an appointment when you call, then the nurse asks you to explain it again, and finally, the doctor wants to rehash the details during your visit. We understand that "vagina" is not a comfortable word for many people and that finding the terms to describe a sexual concern is a challenge for many; however, it is nearly impossible to test or treat someone who won't describe her problem at all.

Frequently, I have blanks next to names in my schedule because a person requested an appointment but would not disclose their concern to the receptionist or the nurse. We can slog through the appointment this way, but it truly is much easier and more efficient for you to state your complaint openly. If you have a "bump down there," we can easily assess this in a quick appointment and have the supplies ready in advance for a biopsy or culture if necessary. If you want to talk about pain with intercourse, you don't need to describe every detail of your sex life to the receptionist; however, stating "I need an appointment because I am experiencing pain with sex," will allow you to be scheduled with enough time for a thorough evaluation of this important problem.

The funny thing is that if you make a big stink about not telling any of the staff why you are in the office, they are then very curious after you leave. Of course, offices don't make overhead announcements that Mary was here for vaginal discharge, and patient confidentiality is of utmost importance; but, as insurance claims are processed, test results are returned, and follow-up appointments are made, the gist of it may become known. People will naturally be much more curious about why you didn't want anyone to know what you came in for than they are about the other 20 patients who came in for the same thing that day. The best approach is to state your concern using appropriate language (go ahead, say "vagina" instead of "hoo hoo," "kitty," or whatever other term you have) in a very matter-of-fact way and I promise, no one will even think twice about it.

23.

I Hate Pap Smears

Everyone hates pap smears. I know, I hear this every day. I have to get one too, and I hate it as much as you do. Even though I collect pap smears all day long, when I find myself sitting naked and freezing on an exam table covered by a paper napkin cruelly disguised as a gown, I feel awkward, sweaty, shy, and uncomfortable. If you feel anxious or uncomfortable about having your pap smear, this means you are totally normal. However, if you want the best care and attention from your provider, I would recommend not repeating over and over how much you hate doctors.

Imagine the service you would receive in a restaurant or hair salon if you marched in, sat down, and stated, "I hate this restaurant," or "I hate people who cut and style hair."

I would never say that, you think.

True, neither would I; however, during gynecology appointments, people routinely march in, sit down, and state: "I haven't had my pap smear in five years because I hate doctors," or some variation on that. I promise, we already know; there is no need to make us feel worse about our chosen profession. Most of us went into this line of work because we enjoy delivering babies, doing surgery, and promoting women's health. I have yet to hear of a student graduating from medical school who proclaimed, "I really love doing pap smears and examining vaginal discharge; I think I'll become a gynecologist."

24.

What Is the First Day of Your Last Menstrual Period?

When you come to the gynecology office for a pap smear, yeast infection, abnormal bleeding, or any other complaint, I am 100 percent certain that you *will* be asked, "What is the first day of your last menstrual period?" It always amazes me that no one ever seems to know the answer to this question, even when they present with a new pregnancy. Common answers to this question that you should avoid are: "I'm on the blue pills in my pill pack," or "My next period is due in a week." There are numerous reasons that gynecologists ask about the first day of your last period, but here are some of the most common:

1. To see if you are late and could be pregnant.

2. If you are newly pregnant, to establish your due date and gestational age.

3. To see if your menstrual cycles are regular.

4. To see if your birth control pills are working as expected.

5. To see if you are at a point in your menstrual cycle when we can order relevant blood tests, ultrasounds, or procedures that may help clarify the issue you are being evaluated for. For example: a dye test often used to evaluate infertile couples can only be done on cycle days 3–7.

If you can, come to your appointment prepared with this information. If you don't know or don't keep track, that means you are totally normal. Most women do not track their menstrual cycles (myself included) unless they are planning a pregnancy. However, knowing you will be asked this question at your appointment will allow you to look at a calendar, look at your pill pack, or use whatever strategy you prefer to figure this out in advance and be prepared when you come to the office. I guarantee that if you can answer this question straight away when asked, you will totally amaze the office nurse...she may even be rendered speechless!

25.

I Forgot I Had That

"What is this huge scar on your chest from?" I asked.

"Oh, that was from my open-heart surgery and quadruple bypass. I forgot I had that."

Kudos to the surgeon who performed such an amazing operation that the patient forgot about her major heart surgery, but this type of past medical history is critical for all providers (including the gynecologist) to be made aware of. Incidentally, this patient, a lovely woman in her mid-50s came in for a pap smear reporting *no* prior surgeries. I noticed the scar during her breast exam!

You can improve the quality of your medical care by knowing your health history or carrying a copy with you. As you probably already realize, every time you visit a new physician's office, you will be asked questions about your current health and your past medical history. Each office will have different forms to complete, but the questions are often similar. A run-of-the-mill health history includes your current medical conditions, prior medical problems, hospitalizations, past surgeries, current medications, drug allergies, family history, pregnancies, and social situation.

If you have a difficult time remembering your medications or have a complex history, consider spending a few hours typing up a list of the basics to bring with you to each new physician appointment. Making sure your chart is correct and up to date can dramatically affect the care you receive. For example, if I don't know you had a blood clot in your leg ten years ago because you forgot, I might prescribe a medication that increases your chances of developing blood clots, which could be life threatening. Having an accurate medical record is also important for billing purposes and the assignment of preexisting conditions (or lack of such) for insurance.

If you feel motivated, use the following outline to create your own standard gynecologic health history.

Name

Age

Occupation

Current medical conditions (examples would be diabetes, cancer in remission, asthma)

Hospitalizations (Have you stayed in the hospital overnight for a reason other than childbirth?)

Past surgeries (examples would be knee replacement, tonsils, appendix, tubal ligation, hysterectomy)

Current medications (include vitamins, herbals, and over-the-counter drugs)

Drug and food allergies (the ones that cause hives, swelling, rash or trouble breathing; not the ones that cause nausea or upset stomach)

Prior sexually transmitted diseases and/or abnormal pap smears

Current method of pregnancy prevention and/or when you went through menopause

General description of your periods (occur every four weeks and last four days with heavy bleeding)

Social habits (Do you smoke, drink, use drugs? Do you feel safe in your relationship? Do you have a place to live?)

Total number of pregnancies and what happened with each one (miscarriage, abortion, vaginal birth, c-section)

Family history (Do your parents or siblings have any major medical conditions or cancer?)

26.

I Had a Red Bump Last Week

If you have a lesion or wart or lump or bump or rash or swelling, you must come into the office when it is *visible* for your doctor to evaluate the area in question. Many people ask, "I had a red bump last week but now it's gone. What do you think that was?" When I can't give a clear explanation, frustration follows. Most clinics have a doctor on call and same-day appointment slots available for patients with acute problems. You will rarely get a same-day appointment for a pap smear (there really is no such thing as an "emergency pap smear"), but, if you have a vaginal rash that suddenly appeared, it is very reasonable to have an immediate evaluation. If, however, you call with a rash that has been present for 3 months and request an appointment immediately, you will probably not be offered one of the same-day slots, because the rash has already been present for some time.

This situation also applies to diagnosis over the phone. Often patients call and ask, "I have an area of redness and burning in my vagina. What do you think is causing it?" Without looking at the area in question, I don't know if it is a cut or scrape, a yeast infection, a herpes outbreak, Lichen Sclerosus (a skin condition), a Bartholin gland abscess, or something else. If you call with this type of symptom, you will generally be advised to come in for an appointment.

It is also prudent to assume that a pelvic exam could be part of every office visit. How would you feel if you went to the cardiologist (heart doctor) reporting chest pain and the doctor didn't listen to your heart with a stethoscope? I am guessing if you went to the cardiologist, you would expect, if not demand, a heart exam. I understand that exposing your vagina under fluorescent lighting to the eyes of a stranger is uncomfortable and embarrassing; however, it is nearly impossible to guess what is causing most gynecologic symptoms when you are fully clothed.

27.

It's Okay to Ask: How Much Will This Cost?

Medical costs are outrageous these days, and a quick office visit for a yeast infection can cost several hundred dollars. I am amazed how often patients agree to tests, procedures, appointments, and the like with no understanding of how much of their hard-earned money it will actually cost. Many assume their insurance will cover the bill, and others assume it won't be much. Understandably, patients often feel that if a test is recommended by their doctor that it is mandatory regardless of cost. Not true. While more information is often better when trying to establish a diagnosis, you should have a clear understanding of what details are expected to be revealed by each test. Feel free to have an open discussion with your doctor about the financial costs and clinical value of the tests or procedures they recommend. Every office should have a staff person who can tell you exactly how much a given appointment or lab will cost. If you have financial concerns, ask in advance, as many things are billed separately.

For example, if you have an office appointment with a physician, an ultrasound, a pap smear, and blood work, these are all separate charges. The office appointment is one charge based on the time your physician spent with you (5, 10, 15, 30, or 60 minutes), or the complexity of the visit. The ultrasound has two separate charges: one technical to collect the images, and one professional to interpret the images as normal or not. The pap smear may have as many as three charges: one from the physician for collecting the pap smear sample, one from the lab for processing, and one from the pathology department for interpreting the processed sample. Finally, the blood work may have two or more charges: one for the sample collection (needle into your arm), and a separate charge for each test run. If you have your thyroid hormone level checked and your cholesterol checked, this will be two separate charges.

Fortunately, most people have insurance that covers many of these costs, but it is unwise to make assumptions about your specific insurance plan. Go ahead, ask how much an ultrasound will cost, and check with your insurance company before proceeding with the test if money is a concern. Unless you are being treated emergently, there is usually plenty of time to investigate potential costs and understand your options.

28.

Have You Done This Before?

I find it utterly shocking that of all the surgeries I have ever performed, only twice in 12 years have I been asked about my surgical experience, even during training when I was doing certain procedures for the very first time! If you are planning a surgery, it is okay to ask, "How many times have you done this?" Your doctor will not be offended. Let's face it, someone is going to cut into your body with a knife; this is serious and important. You want expertise. You want to feel confident that your doctor knows what he or she is doing.

Oddly enough, people often judge their doctor's surgical skills based on personality. This is totally different from surgical expertise. A nice person with excellent bedside manner may, in fact, be a terrible surgeon! Fortunately, most of us are skilled and competent at the procedures we advise. If not, we often bring as our surgical assistant another physician who has more experience to supervise. Both of these arrangements are totally acceptable and routine. What you don't want is someone who does a given procedure *rarely*, operating alone. Go ahead, ask your doctor: "Have you done this before? How many times? When was the most recent time you performed this operation? Do you feel comfortable with this procedure? Who will your assistant be?" Here are a few other important questions to ask your surgeon:

1. What are the risks and potential complications of this procedure?

2. Have you had any patients with complications during surgery?

3. What limitations will I have after this procedure?

4.   What other questions should I be asking about this procedure or diagnosis? (This is probably the most important question you could ask).

Also, be absolutely certain that you actually read and understand what is written on your surgical consent form. The form should *not* read "I consent to the following procedure: TAH, BSO." Do you really know what a TAH, BSO is? I see this all the time. Instead of "TAH, BSO," the consent form should read something along the lines of: "Remove uterus, cervix, and ovaries through open-belly surgery." This makes sense, and the planned procedure is clearly described. If the form you are being asked to sign does not make sense to you, speak up; it can and should be rewritten.

Finally, be sure you understand what outcome and side effects to expect after surgery. In medical school, I remember observing a meeting between a surgeon and his patient following a hysterectomy. The patient asked her doctor if she would be able to have more children...*after* he had just removed her uterus. Clearly, there was a communication breakdown prior to surgery. It should have been very clear to this woman that following the surgical removal of her uterus, she would not be able to have more children. Don't become an example in my next book...ask anything and everything that is on your mind.

29.

Doctor, Do I Have Cancer?

Over the years, I have become better and better at guessing what is really bothering someone based on reported symptoms; however, much of the time I am still really far off. As healers, doctors want to address your concerns. We want to reassure you, but as scientific types, we are poor intuitive guessers. Because we lack Jedi minds, I encourage you to openly discuss with your doctor what you are really concerned about. This means if you are worried that you have cancer, please say so. If you are scared your IUD (intrauterine device) is causing infertility, speak up. Often, women present to the office with a stated problem such as: "I have bad cramps with my periods," which is *not* their true concern (that they have uterine cancer because Aunt Susan was recently diagnosed). I spend the entire appointment ignorantly yammering on about causes of menstrual cramps and possible solutions. The distraught patient subsequently leaves my office feeling completely unheard because I didn't mentioned uterine cancer; meanwhile, I feel I have solved her problem with menstrual cramps.

I believe that patients don't mention their true concerns because they worry that the physician will think their question is stupid, their concern is frivolous, or they will find out that you searched the Internet prior to your appointment. Even if you did consult Dr. Google, don't worry. If you are certain that your symptoms mean cancer and your doctor doesn't mention this, ask him directly: "I'm scared. Do my symptoms mean cancer?" If you are worried you can never have sex again because you have HPV (human papillomavirus), let us know. Most concerns are easily allayed if we know exactly what they are. Incidentally, IUDs do not cause infertility (I have known more than one woman who conceived the same day her IUD was removed), menstrual cramps do not mean uterine cancer, and yes, you can have sex again if you have been diagnosed with HPV.

30.

Understand ALL Your Treatment Options

Did your mother have a hysterectomy? This means you will need one too, right? Actually, you should know that there are often multiple ways to treat a given problem. For example, let's say you are 42 years old and bleeding every two weeks. Years ago, your only treatment option might have been hysterectomy (surgical removal of the uterus). Today, your treatment options might include: (1) no treatment, (2) Depo-Provera injections, (3) oral contraceptive pills, (4) a Mirena IUD, (5) NovaSure ablation, or (6) hysterectomy.

Many women still believe that if they experience abnormal bleeding, a hysterectomy is the only treatment option. If such a person meets with a physician who loves to operate, she may end up with a hysterectomy costing thousands of dollars and with six weeks off work when a Mirena IUD placed during an office visit would have solved the bleeding problem. Ask your doctor what *all* your options are, and ask her to explain why she is recommending a given treatment. Ultimately, the physician should offer you a list of options with associated risks and benefits and then let you decide how to proceed.

Another example of a condition with several treatment options is depressed mood. Believe it or not, medication is far from the only solution for depressive symptoms. Many women request "that pill I saw on TV" or, are reluctant to talk with their doctors at all about depression because they assume prescription medication is the only option. Other possible treatments for depression include aerobic exercise, individual or couples counseling, dietary and lifestyle modifications, Vitamin D supplementation, and acupuncture. Feel free to ask your doctor, "What other options do I have? What will happen if I do nothing? Why are you recommending this strategy versus what I saw on TV or what my friend takes?" For more information on stress and depression, or to speak with a holistic health coach about this issue, visit www.RedLetterHealth.com.

31.

Menopause Is Puberty in Reverse

Do you remember going through puberty? If you are like me, thoughts of puberty do not bring pleasant memories to mind. I remember being covered in pimples, feeling moody and irritable, and having a number of physical symptoms I did not like and did not understand. Somewhere between age 12 and age 20, both my mind and my body went through a lot of changes. I felt physically and emotionally different at age 8 than I did at age 20.

Puberty is a time of increasing hormones. You have *low* hormones before puberty; there is an *increase* with associated symptoms during puberty, and then a new steady state of *high* hormones when puberty maturation is complete. In menopause, the opposite occurs. You have *high* hormones before menopause; there is a *decline* over several years with associated symptoms, and then a new steady state of *low* hormones develops when menopause is complete (average age is around 52). Some women have an easy time of both puberty and menopause, whereas others suffer greatly.

The menopause transition is part of normal aging in the same way that puberty is part of normal aging. Nothing bad is happening. You will feel symptoms including hot flashes, vaginal dryness, decline in libido, night sweats, changes in memory and concentration, dry skin, mood swings, and the like (sounds awful, right?). This is comparable to the increased libido, acne, body odor, hair growth, and emotional disturbances you likely experienced during puberty. Your doctor can help you manage the symptoms of menopause with diet, lifestyle, and hormonal treatments if needed; however, the symptoms themselves are to be expected. Contrary to popular belief, most women do not need to take hormones during the menopause transition.

Following the menopause transition, you will reach a new steady state of low hormones that will continue from your mid-50s through the rest of your life. It is not necessary to check your hormone levels in menopause to see if they are low, because they *are* naturally low. We would not expect a lady in menopause to have the hormone levels of a 30-year-old any more than we would expect a six-year-old to have those levels. I see many menopausal women for the concern of "low hormones" and they are shocked to find out it is true and natural and, in fact, not a disease to be cured with drugs or surgery. If you are experiencing bothersome symptoms during menopause, talk openly with your doctor about how you feel and learn what options are available for relief.

32.

There Are No Hormones in Your Tubes or Uterus.

Hormones are produced by organs such as your ovaries, adrenal glands, thyroid, and brain. Your tubes are basically conduits for eggs, sperm, and early embryos. Fallopian tubes do not produce hormones and your uterus is a very specialized container for a baby to grow. The uterus typically does not produce hormones either. I know I am going to sound outrageous here but, since there are no hormones in your fallopian tubes, if you have your "tubes tied," you are not going to experience hormone changes after surgery. "Tying" the tubes simply means that you are disconnecting the passageway between the ovaries and the uterus so the egg cannot meet the sperm, thereby preventing pregnancy. Even after your tubes are tied the ovary continues to function normally, and still produces a microscopic egg every month that is reabsorbed by the body.

Similarly, women often avoid hysterectomy (surgical removal of the uterus) even when medically indicated because they fear the effect it will have on their hormones. I have had women who bleed so excessively each month that they require blood transfusions refuse hysterectomy in fear that their hormones will be altered. As long as your ovaries are left untouched, you should not notice dramatic hormonal changes after hysterectomy.

In contrast, I have known women to request hysterectomy because they are "bitchy" during their periods or because they experience severe PMS. They feel that if they don't bleed regularly, they will notice improved hormones and improved mood. Removing the uterus alone will not improve mood other than to relieve the annoyance of bleeding every month. As long as you have ovaries and are not yet in menopause (average age of menopause is 52), you will still experience PMS symptoms, including mood swings, every 28 days or so. Removing the uterus permanently ends uterine bleeding, decreases pelvic pain and pressure in some cases, and eliminates the possibility of pregnancy…that's it.

33.

Opinions on Hormones

Taking hormones of any kind is highly controversial. Some people won't eat meat because of potential hormone contamination, while others take handfuls of hormone pills every day. Just as individual women have strong opinions on the safety and efficacy of hormone treatments, individual doctors have the same. You can imagine how the visit goes if you are a person who takes handfuls of hormone supplements and you are meeting with a doctor who is totally opposed to all hormones. Likewise, you can imagine the conflict if you are avoiding meat to avoid hormones and your doctor advises progesterone injections for contraception or fertility.

Although there are a few standard guidelines for hormone therapy, most doctors prescribe or advise hormones based on their personal beliefs. Don't assume that the doctor you are seeing has the same opinions you do about hormones. Here are some current basic guidelines that most western medical physicians follow:

1. Birth control pills are safe unless you have a contraindication. (Some common contraindications include being a smoker over age 35, having a personal history of migraine with aura, having personal or family history of a blood clot, having personal history of breast cancer, and having uncontrolled high blood pressure).

2. Hormone therapy for menopause symptoms is to be used for the shortest period of time in the lowest dose to manage intolerable symptoms of menopause (hot flashes, vaginal dryness, night sweats, etc.)—up to five years and then discontinued. It is not meant to be used

forever. I know, your 83-year-old aunt still takes estrogen, but this is not a standard recommendation.

3. Most women do not *need* hormone replacement during menopause. Hormone replacement is only for those women who experience such intolerable symptoms that they cannot function normally. For example, their hot flashes may be so severe that they cannot concentrate at work or drive a car.

4. Bioidentical hormones, hormones compounded in a pharmacy, or hormone preparations purchased over-the-counter are not safer than traditional pharmaceutical hormones. They are all hormones. Period.

5. The only reason to test a person's hormone levels is if a hormone-producing tumor is suspected. This is rare. If you are having regular menstrual cycles, your hormones are generally normal (including thyroid). If you are in menopause (12 months with no period around the age of 52), your hormones are low across the board, and you do not need a test to identify this. Menopause is a natural state of low hormones and is part of normal aging. The goal of hormone therapy is to help you manage intolerable symptoms during the menopause transition, not to bring your hormones up to their pre-menopause level.

With this information in mind, realize that some physicians are strong supporters of bioidentical hormones and will gladly test your saliva or blood hormone levels and prescribe them liberally. Other physicians are totally opposed and will try at every appointment to talk you out of the hormone therapy you have been on for years. There are many physicians with many opinions on this controversial topic. To find a provider aligned with your personal beliefs, ask when you schedule your appointment if the physician you are seeing is willing to prescribe the hormone treatment that you want, or if they are willing to order hormone tests at your request. Knowing your doctor's stance on hormone therapies in menopause prior to your appointment can save you time, money, and allow you to meet with someone who shares your views.

34.

Your Hormones Are Probably Normal

"My husband thinks there is something wrong with me. I'm not interested in sex. He thinks I need my hormones checked." I hear this in my office at least once a day. Unfortunately, there is no laboratory test to assess low libido or any other perceived hormone problem including mood swings and irritability. Here is an easy test you can do at home: Ask yourself if you are having a menstrual period roughly every four to five weeks or so. If the answer is yes, your hormones are most likely normal.

While I truly do wish the situation were different, birth control pills won't change your bad relationship. Testosterone patches won't morph your spouse into Brad Pitt. Wild-yam creams won't make your thighs smaller. Progesterone won't vaporize your mother-in-law. And estrogen patches won't give you a kinder boss. Many reported "hormone" problems are actually "life" problems and no amount of supplements will make a difference. That being said, I have known women who swear that progesterone cream saved their marriage, while others felt it made no difference whatsoever. My best advice: talk with your doctor openly about what you are experiencing; he or she will likely be able to help you feel better, even if the solution is not hormonal. If you prefer to take compounded hormone supplements at any age, I would encourage you to consider meeting with a naturopathic physician, or visiting an endocrinologist (a western medical doctor who specializes in hormone imbalances).

Here are some general truths about hormones:

1.   If you are having regular menstrual cycles (roughly once a month), your hormones (including thyroid) are likely

fine. Your menstrual cycle will often be the first to go if your hormones are out of whack.

2.   There is a natural decline in hormone levels during menopause. Please see the sections of this book titled "Menopause Is Puberty in Reverse" and "Opinions on Hormones" for more information on this topic.

3.   The average age of menopause is 52. If you are 32 years old and reporting hot flashes, it is not likely to be early menopause.

35.

Pills versus Pregnancy

Be smart about hormonal contraception and blood clots. Many women tell me that they don't want to use hormonal contraception (oral contraceptive pills, Mirena IUD, Depo-Provera, NuvaRing, Ortho Evra patch) because they are worried about blood clots. Most often, this is something learned from advertisements listing risks on TV.

While it is true that taking certain hormones can increase your risk of blood clots, did you know that your chances of developing a blood clot are also increased during pregnancy? In fact, you are more likely to develop a blood clot during pregnancy than while taking any type of hormonal contraception. If you don't use a reliable method of pregnancy prevention, you can become unexpectedly pregnant and your chances of a clot are increased at that time. If you prefer not to use hormonal contraception, that is totally acceptable, as many women prefer alternative methods (including condoms and Paraguard IUD), but always keep in mind that you are more likely to develop a blood clot while pregnant than while on birth control pills.

This line of thinking also applies to birth control pills and weight gain. Although most people don't gain weight on birth control pills, they typically do gain 30 to 50 pounds while pregnant. Avoiding hormonal contraception to avoid weight gain and then becoming unintentionally pregnant (and gaining 50 lbs) seems convoluted. When considering the risks of contraceptive options, including birth control pills, remember to compare your preferences to the risk of unplanned pregnancy.

Incidentally, if you prefer to use a non-hormonal method of birth control such as natural family planning, be sure you understand how this is done. Counting forward 14 days from the first day of your last period and avoiding intercourse around that time is absolutely incorrect! The only way to know for certain when you ovulated (produced an egg) and are fertile, is to count *backwards* 14 days from the start of your period. Seem confusing? It is. Be sure to keep a menstrual calendar for at least 3 months and discuss your cycles in detail with your doctor prior to counting on natural family planning as a reliable means of preventing pregnancy.

36.

Doctor Google

What you see on television is marketing, not medicine. There it is again, that commercial with the happy smiling people, showing you how great your life will be if you only take a given medication. They all say, "Talk to your doctor to see if this medication is right for you," but what they really mean is that you should ask your doctor to prescribe this for you. I can't tell you the number of people who have a symptom of some kind, diagnose themselves with a given condition by searching the Internet, and then determine that a drug they saw on a TV commercial is the right solution. By the time they come to my office, they no longer want to discuss their symptoms or consider a diagnosis; they only want me to write a prescription for the drug they saw to treat their self-diagnosed condition. It is nearly impossible to talk these people out of the drug they have decided on or out of the diagnosis they have established in a Google search.

Doctors do prescribe medications, but we are not pill dispensers. Some days, I wonder why I even bother to go to work, given that seemingly all conditions can be diagnosed and treated by Dr. Google and TV. I encourage you to search the Internet for your symptoms, talk with people, and collect information but always keep an open mind during your medical evaluation. What you do or don't actually have could differ greatly from what you came up with on your own.

Believe me; I understand this tendency, as I experienced it with my dog. Baker had several months' worth of itchy skin and was scratching day and night, driving me insane. My Google search yielded a diagnosis of food allergy. I took him to the vet, and she prescribed antibiotics for a skin staph infection, which I didn't give him initially because I believed it was a food allergy. I thought my two days of Internet research and a discussion with a lady in PetSmart were clearly more accurate than my vet's years of training and experience. I changed his food several times with no improvement. After weeks of more scratching, I finally gave him the antibiotics just to prove the vet was incorrect, and to my surprise, Baker got instantly better. No more scratching; so much for my theory of food allergy.

37.

Is the Pain in Your Left Lower Belly?

Most of us carry around ten or more pounds of stagnant poop in our intestines—gross! Did you know that left lower belly pain is almost always caused by your intestine, not your ovary? In your left lower belly, your large intestine (colon) makes an S-shaped turn (the sigmoid colon) before it empties into the rectum. This area often becomes clogged with constipation in the same way the S-shaped turns of the various drains in your house can become clogged. When there is a backlog of poop in the sigmoid colon, your left lower belly hurts. Sometimes, you can even feel the hard poop as a solid lump in your left lower belly.

Naturally, when feeling a lump or experiencing pain in the left lower belly, most women believe it is an ovarian problem. They worry they have an ovarian cyst or ovarian cancer. Fortunately, this is almost never the case. Instead, most women are chronically constipated. This is generally a result of diet (not enough fresh fruits and veggies, too much processed food, meat, and dairy) and insufficient plain water intake (at least 32 ounces per day). Do you have a bowel movement at least once per day? Did you know that constipation is a risk factor for colon cancer? Moving your bowels is critical to good health and also leads to a flatter belly. What woman do you know who doesn't want a flatter belly?! Here are some dietary suggestions for colon health:

1. Consume a tablespoon of flaxseed oil once per day.

2. Add flaxseeds or flaxseed oil to salad, juice, or smoothies.

3. Increase your intake of fresh fruits and vegetables. Ideally, this should make up about 50% of your daily food intake.

4. Use quinoa as a grain in any recipe that calls for rice.

5. Add beets to salads or roasted vegetable dishes, or drink fresh beet juice (actually very sweet).

6. Drink at least 32 oz of plain water per day.

7. Cut down on caffeine and alcohol, both of which can actually be dehydrating. Caffeine is also a stimulant to the intestine and can act as a laxative, but as with all stimulant laxatives, chronic use can make your intestinal function dependent on this to move.

8. Cut down on processed foods and heavy meats as these move very slowly through the intestine.

38.

Are You a Medical Mystery?

Fortunately, it is very unlikely that you are a medical mystery. Many women report they "don't feel well" and are certain "there is something wrong." They are convinced they have cancer, a rare disease, or an unusual and mysterious condition that no one can diagnose. Their blood tests and physical exams are normal, and yet they still feel crappy. They often seek several opinions from several providers and have no diagnosis. This is frustrating for both the patient and provider. I have had patients with this situation go to Mayo Clinic and pay for flights, hotel rooms, and hundreds of tests only to be told they are "normal," unfortunately leaving more frustrated than when they arrived.

When something feels wrong with your body, it is natural to feel scared and jump to worst case scenarios; however, more commonly, people don't feel physically well because of dietary choices, lack of exercise, stress, strained relationships, unfulfilling careers, and lack of purpose or meaning in life. These conditions are not diagnosable with CT scans or blood tests and are generally not treated with medications. Many people also have sensitivities to caffeine, gluten, soy, dairy, meat, sugar, or other foods. I know many women who have eliminated processed foods and sugar from their diets only to discover that they not only feel ten years younger but that numerous medical conditions have inexplicably vanished! Food sensitivity testing is becoming more and more popular amongst both patients and physicians and is something to consider if you have undiagnosed symptoms.

Also, dehydration is often the source of many bothersome conditions, and simply scrapping the caffeine and/or alcohol, and drinking more water can solve a variety of problems. For me personally, simply drinking water healed years of chronic daily headaches, dry skin, acne, knee pain, back muscle spasms, and it dramatically improved my mood. Many people are also deficient in basic vitamins such as Vitamin D (which can affect immune system and mood). Lack of exercise can lead to decreased energy, lymph stagnation, depressed mood, and poor self-image. You don't need to train for a marathon, but even a ten-minute walk outdoors can make a huge difference in how you feel. Additionally, if you hate your job or are in a career that is misaligned with your personal values, it's no wonder you have terrible belly pain or migraines on Monday mornings. Did you know most heart attacks occur on Monday mornings? If you are struggling in your relationship, it is no wonder you are not interested in sex.

Yes, you may certainly have a serious or elusive medical condition (such as Lyme disease) and I encourage you to search vigilantly, seek consultations, and have comprehensive medical testing; but, as you search for explanations, also consider your own diet, lifestyle, relationships, and career for clues as to why you might be feeling unwell. Incidentally, if you have healed yourself of a seemingly mysterious illness or incurable symptom, your success story might help others. You may be perfectly suited for a career in holistic health coaching. If this interests you, visit RedLetterHealth.com for more information.

39.

Your Real Blood Pressure

Your blood pressure in the doctor's office is probably your real blood pressure. I know you are anxious about your pap smear. No one wants to get undressed (including me) for their pap smear or gynecologic exam. It's embarrassing and uncomfortable; however, the anxiety you feel about this is unlikely to raise your blood pressure out of the normal range. You wouldn't believe the list of excuses I hear for high blood pressure. A patient will be in my office with a pressure of 200/120 (normal is under 140/90) stating her blood pressure is unusually high because "I just walked up the stairs," "My nephew crashed the car yesterday," "I'm nervous about my appointment," "I hate the gynecologist," "I drank five cups of coffee this morning," and on and on and on.

If walking up stairs and drinking coffee raise your blood pressure to a dangerous level, you still have a serious problem. And although you might be anxious at your appointment, your blood pressure still should not be excessively high. The so-called "white-coat hypertension" at the doctor's office should not raise your blood pressure to the level of a possible stroke! People also often state: "I've never had a high blood pressure in the past," while their medical record from prior appointments reveals a different story.

It's perplexing that we are so resistant to accepting that our blood pressures may be elevated. Personally, I want to know if my blood pressure is elevated so I can tackle this problem immediately. I don't want to develop kidney problems, heart disease, vision issues, or, most especially, stroke because I ignored my blood pressure. This condition is easily treated most commonly with diet and lifestyle changes and sometimes medication. If your blood pressure is up at your appointment, I encourage you to embrace and tackle this issue instead of reciting a list of reasons why you think it is falsely high or of falling victim to denial. It could save your life.

The same is true for height and weight. More than half the time, when these parameters are checked in the office, patients report "I shrunk two inches since last year!" or "My scale at home says I weigh 30 lbs less." It's amazing that these measurements in my office are wrong for so many patients! Incidentally, while some height loss is common with normal aging, if you truly have shrunk two inches in one year, you may need a bone density test.

40.

Assume You Are Vitamin D Deficient

Do you expose roughly half your naked body to direct sunlight (not through a window) for 20 minutes per day without sunscreen? If not you are probably vitamin D deficient. Vitamin D is important for bone strength, brain function, mood, and immune function. This vitamin is primarily synthesized in the skin after direct sunlight exposure. It is also found in foods such as cod liver oil and sardines. People with darker skin have more difficulty synthesizing vitamin D because of the protective effect of the dark pigment in the skin. This means those with darker skin require even more exposure to sunlight to manufacture vitamin D naturally within their bodies.

As a physician in Montana where, we rarely expose our skin to sunlight, I have seen many people with Vitamin D deficiency. Supplementing with a liquid or gel formulation of Vitamin D3 of 1000 to 2000 units daily has helped me personally tackle depressed mood in the winter months and has also helped countless numbers of my patients feel generally better. Your doctor can order a blood test to tell if you are deficient in vitamin D. A good target level is between 50 and 90 ng/mL, with 30 ng/mL being the lowest acceptable blood level. I have found in my practice that most people begin to feel better once their levels are above 50 ng/mL. Ask your doctor if a blood test for vitamin D or a vitamin supplement might benefit you, especially if you suffer from generally depressed mood or fatigue.

41.

Don't Expect an Orgasm during Sex

What? I thought the whole purpose of having sex was to experience orgasm! Why would anyone have sex otherwise? Some of you are reading this and feeling outraged while others are feeling relieved. How do I know? Day after day, a few brave women muster the courage to ask me about sex during their medical appointment or pap smear. They want to know what is wrong with them because they have to "fake it" every time or they have never had an orgasm during sexual intercourse. Here's a secret: the female vagina is analogous to the male *scrotum.* Stimulating a woman's vagina is akin to stimulating a man's scrotum. It might feel good for both parties but is unlikely to generate an orgasm for either one. The male penis is analogous to the female clitoris and this area usually requires direct stimulation for orgasm. The bottom line is that many women do not get adequate stimulation of the clitoris during vaginal intercourse and therefore don't orgasm. Nothing is wrong here, there is just a simple lack of anatomical understanding unfortunately, perpetuated by mainstream media.

On TV and movies Hollywood stars always orgasm together in the midst of passionate sex. While this is certainly possible, it is far from the norm. Given the differences between male and female anatomy as well as the differences in timing of the sexual response cycle for both genders (shorter and linear for men, longer and variable for women), it is unusual to experience what you see on TV with your partner. A more common experience is for each person to orgasm sequentially with different types of physical stimulation; this means taking turns. He does what works for you, and you do what works for him. Open discussion about sexual issues with both your doctor and your partner will make for a much more satisfying sex life. Faking it eventually leads to boredom and dissatisfaction for the woman, and can ruin your relationship if and when he finds out he is not the stud in the bedroom that you made him think he was. Faking orgasm or sexual enjoyment is also lying to your partner which does not make for a solid relationship regardless of circumstance.

The good news is that usually an open discussion, an anatomy lesson, and a little experimentation in the bedroom can lead to fun and enjoyable sexual interactions and orgasms for everyone! Don't be shy about asking your doctor about all your sexual concerns (remember as gynecologists we have already heard and won't judge what you are about to ask) and try not to criticize yourself or your partner if you have not yet experienced orgasm. Find the courage and the language to ask your doctor about sex and you won't be disappointed.

42.

My Breasts Are Lumpy

All women have lumpy breasts. These lumps are the fat and glandular tissues that create normal breasts. The glands might swell and change at various times during your menstrual cycle, during pregnancy, or while you are breast-feeding. The idea behind breast self-exam is not for you to become a master clinician but rather, for you to get a sense of what your breasts normally feel like and to note any new lumps or changes that aren't typically there. This can easily be done in the shower as follows: Lift your arm over your head and feel your breast for five or ten seconds while washing. If you do this every time you shower, chances are, you will notice what the normal glandular cycles are for your breasts as well as the presence of any new lumps. The lumps you are checking for might feel like stones or rubbery pencil erasers. If you notice something new, get a checkup immediately. Another thing you can easily watch for is skin dimpling or clumping on the skin over your breast. Again, if you notice this, get a checkup immediately. Finally, some yellowish or whitish discharge from your nipple is normal, especially if you squeeze your breast or are pregnant or nursing. If you see bloody nipple discharge, however, get a checkup immediately.

Regarding mammograms, current guidelines advise a mammogram every year after age 40. The idea behind mammograms is that they can detect a breast cancer much earlier than a clinical breast exam. This means that by the time you feel a lump (if it is cancer), it can be a much more advanced stage than something microscopic detected via mammogram. The cancerous lump that you found or that I felt in the office might require mastectomy (removal of the whole breast), chemotherapy, and radiation to treat, whereas the microscopic cancer found by mammogram might require only lumpectomy (a small amount of tissue removed from the breast) to be cured.

Women are often fearful of mammograms, and no one wants to experience the temporary discomfort of having their breast squished (including me), but a mammogram could save your life. I am frequently asked: "What if the mammogram causes breast cancer with radiation?" The bottom line is that mammograms can detect *early* cancer, as I described above, and, I once read that the radiation you receive from a mammogram is about the same as the radiation you receive from flying across the US in a commercial airplane. Be sure to discuss your concerns about mammograms with your doctor so you can learn the facts about this important cancer screening tool and don't worry if your breasts always feel generally lumpy. As a doctor, one way I know if a woman has had breast implants is if I feel smooth, symmetrical tissue instead of generally lumpy tissue under the skin during my exam.

43.

It's Okay Not to Bleed

Monthly menstrual bleeding is a funny thing. Some women are happy to see their period every month because it makes them feel normal. If they don't see one, they believe the uterine lining is building up inside of them and a toxic mass of cells is about to blow! Other women feel cursed by their monthly cycle and will go to great lengths, including major surgery, to get rid of it. The truth is, there are many situations in which it is perfectly okay not to bleed every month.

Some examples of situations in which it is safe not to bleed monthly include the presence of a Mirena IUD inside your uterus, the use of oral contraceptive (birth control) pills, the use of Depo Provera injections, or the use of Implanon for contraception. Some women do not bleed regularly while breastfeeding, and skipped cycles are also common in the early teens and late 40s when menstrual hormones are ramping up and slowing down, respectively. Women who are receiving chemotherapy and women who are extremely underweight may also not experience monthly periods.

If you do not fall into any of the categories that I listed above, and you are not having cyclic bleeding approximately every 21-35 days, consult with your doctor as to what the cause might be, especially if you are planning a pregnancy. If, however, you want to use a Mirena IUD to prevent pregnancy, don't worry about the possible side effect of not bleeding. In this case, the uterine lining is actually very *thin*, and excess menstrual blood is *not* getting backlogged inside your body. Talk openly with your doctor about your questions surrounding this topic as it is one of the most common sources of confusion I encounter in my office.

44.

Obesity Is a Health Problem

Really, the only difference between high cholesterol, high blood pressure, and high weight is that only one of these (weight) is visible. No one can look at you and tell if you have dangerously high blood pressure, or a dangerous virus like HIV or hepatitis, but everyone can see who has dangerously high weight. Because this problem is visible, it is perceived as a cosmetic problem; however, weight is really a critical measure of health. Did you know women who are overweight or obese have higher chances of heart attacks, heart disease, diabetes, breast cancer, uterine cancer, and many, many, many, other conditions? During pregnancy, being overweight or obese increases your chances of delivering by cesarean section.

Unfortunately, obese women are treated very poorly in today's society. At a medical conference I recently attended on weight management, the speaker reported that obese women are more discriminated against and loathed in American society than any other race, ethnicity, or political group. He described a study showing a thin woman going into a store and being treated kindly and then the same woman going back into the same store a few minutes later wearing a fat suit and being treated awfully. I find this very disturbing and wonder how many thin people would be judged if they had to wear their blood pressure readings or their medical conditions including sexually transmitted infections around their necks for all to see.

The good news is that your doctor may be able to help you lower your weight to a level that is both safe for your health and more cosmetically acceptable. Many medical strategies are available today to lower weight including surgery, appetite suppression medications, meal replacement, lifestyle support, and behavior counseling. Different doctors may suggest different strategies so be sure to find a provider who offers a strategy that resonates with you. Ideally, you should find something that works within the context of your busy life and has built-in support to help you sustain a normal weight long term. Of course there are many fad diets and quick fixes on the market and these can generate rapid weight loss; however, most of the time after quick weight loss comes quick weight gain and disappointment. Imagine how ridiculous it would be if you had a dangerously high blood pressure and your doctor advised a program that lowered it for two months and then allowed it to return to the original high level.

The bottom line is, don't be offended if your doctor asks about your weight and what you are doing to address your size. This means they care about your health more than cosmetics and are willing to help you tackle your weight medically. Wouldn't you be worried if your body temperature was elevated to 104 degrees at your appointment and your doctor didn't even acknowledge it was high? Work with your doctor to find a weight management solution that is right and safe for you. Personally, I love facilitating life and health transformations through weight loss and I feel weight management is one of the most rewarding areas of medicine.

45.

Are You Allergic to Toilet Paper?

Contact irritants are a common cause of vulvar and vaginal discomfort. What is a contact irritant? A contact irritant is anything that comes in contact with your skin—in this case, your vulva or vagina. Women often report itching or irritation and are convinced they have a horrible infection when, in fact, they are allergic to their underwear. The most common contact irritants are pantyliners, douche, lubricant, Vagisil, feminine wash, feminine spray, spermicide, condoms, erotic warming gel, soap, body wash, perfume, flavored gel, fabric softener, and laundry detergent. While thankfully, not everyone is sensitive to these products, anything that comes into contact with the genital area can be a source of irritation. Additionally, many women are allergic to certain fabrics, including those in their underwear and pants. I even knew one woman who was allergic to her couch. Towels and sheets washed with certain detergents or fabric softeners can also be the culprit. Also consider swimsuits, toilet paper, bubble bath, tampons, shaving cream, razors, wax preparations, yeast creams, and hot tubs.

If you have vaginal or vulvar irritation, a good strategy is to start with a visit to your doctor to test for infection *before* you self-treat. If an infection is found and treated, great; if not, consider your environment. Eliminate fabric softeners and dryer sheets. Do not apply any products to the area, including soap. Wash with only warm water. Be a detective and ask yourself what is coming into contact with this area. For example, one of my patients narrowed it down to the toilet paper at her job, and another to her new pants. It truly could be anything. Also, over-the-counter products designed to "soothe" irritation often make it worse, especially if there are already abrasions or if the skin is already inflamed.

Additionally, I encourage you to consider that your "yeast infection" could be a sexually transmitted disease such as chlamydia or herpes. Many women self-treat with over-the-counter products for weeks with no improvement. Then they call and request a yeast treatment such as oral Diflucan over the phone. Sometimes your doctor will prescribe a treatment over the phone, but generally, a true yeast infection will resolve with over-the-counter preparations such as Monistat 7 cream. If your "yeast infection" is not going away, visit the office and get tested for other infections. I know it couldn't possibly be chlamydia because you have been married for 20 years, but I see sexually transmitted infections in seemingly low-risk women all the time.

46.

Surprise!

"We are being careful" is not a contraceptive plan. If you don't have a pregnancy prevention strategy, you are planning a pregnancy. Period. At each visit to the gynecology office, you are likely to be asked what strategy you are using to prevent pregnancy. This could be condoms, pills, abstinence, vasectomy, IUD, natural family planning, etc, (note "pulling out" is not a pregnancy-prevention strategy). If, however, you are not using a strategy to prevent pregnancy, we assume you are planning a pregnancy or that if you become pregnant, you will not be surprised.

I am always amazed by the number of women who are not using any pregnancy prevention strategy and yet are shocked when the test is positive. In this day and age with so many good contraceptive options, talk with your doctor about one that will truly work for you and is suited to your lifestyle. There is no reason for "surprise" pregnancy if you have a good prevention strategy. Also, if you are not using some form of reliable pregnancy prevention, please be sure you are avoiding alcohol, drugs, and tobacco and are taking a prenatal vitamin with 800 micrograms of folate (this lowers your chances of having a baby with spina bifida) daily. Also be sure you are not taking medications such as Accutane or Coumadin that could cause birth defects.

Remember that you can become pregnant as long as you are having periods. Many women tell me they are not using contraception because "I'm too old," or "I just had a baby," or "I'm too thin," or "I'm not married." Not true. Realistically, the fact that you just had a baby suggests that you most certainly can become pregnant! If you are 46 years old and having menstrual periods, you can get pregnant...just ask my 46 year old new mom if this is possible! Once you enter menopause (12 months with no period, occurs around the average age of 52), then it is true, you are too old to get pregnant without advanced fertility treatments. The best plan for all women is to use a rock-solid pregnancy prevention strategy that suits your lifestyle unless you are planning a pregnancy.

47.

Consider Regret When Considering Sterilization

Regret is a common side effect of permanent sterilization. This means if you have your tubes tied, especially at a young age, you may regret it. I don't mean to be negative, but consider your decision in light of possible future circumstances, including death, divorce, or tragic accident. No one wants to consider that they may get divorced and take up with a new partner who has no kids and wants a family. No one wants to consider that their spouse could die in an accident and they may marry a new partner who has no kids and wants a family. And certainly, no one wants to consider that something tragic may happen to their current children and they may want to eventually have more.

I wouldn't be saying this if I didn't have so many women sitting in my office with their tubes tied, asking me what they can do to have more children now that their life circumstances are different. Yes, a tubal ligation reversal procedure exists; however, there is no guarantee that because the tubes are reconnected, they will function properly. Also, this procedure can cost $10,000 or more out of pocket, as it is not generally covered by insurance. In vitro fertilization (IVF) is also an alternative but is equally expensive and not generally covered by insurance.

Think carefully about your decision if you are considering permanent sterilization, and realize that permanent means no more babies ever—never, no matter what, not "no more babies until I change my mind five years from now." Also remember that the younger you are when you have your tubes tied, the higher the chances of unplanned pregnancy (or tubal ligation failure) later in life. Approximately 1 in 200 women will become pregnant after having a tubal ligation.

48.

Expect a Pregnancy Test

If you come to your appointment and report that your period occurred over a month ago, unless you are menopausal (12 months with no period around the age of 52), a pregnancy test will be done. Yes, I know you are not sexually active, but people lie. I know you don't lie, but other people do. I can't tell you the number of women who have had positive pregnancy tests in my office and swore they did not have sex. How did this happen? I don't know. What I do know is that if you report a missed period, I will do a pregnancy test no matter what else you say unless you specifically refuse to have one.

Incidentally, the pregnancy tests we have in the doctor's office are essentially the same as the ones in the store. If you had a positive or negative test at home, you are likely to have the same result in the physician's office. Everyone knows someone who had a false positive or negative test, but this is actually very rare. If you took five tests at home and they were all positive, you're pregnant. Also remember, when testing for possible pregnancy, you must test *after* your missed period. Most tests will not be positive until 2–3 weeks after conception, which is generally 5–7 days after your missed period. You cannot test the day after you had sex to see if you conceived the night before.

49.

Not Your Mother's IUD

I get questions every day about IUDs, so here is the skinny: An IUD, aka IUC (intrauterine contraception), is a small T-shaped piece of plastic that sits inside the uterus and prevents pregnancy. I like to call it "no-brain contraception" because, unlike pills, patches, shots, or condoms, you don't have to remember anything. While IUDs are becoming more and more popular, some women are afraid to get one because of a horror story they heard from their mothers or grandmothers. It is true; there were some dangerous problems with former versions of IUDs from years ago, including infection and damage to the uterine wall. The IUDs of today are not your grandmother's IUD, however. They are generally safe and effective.

The two types of IUDs available today are Paraguard (works via copper, good for ten years) and Mirena (works via progesterone, good for five years). Paraguard is the most common form of contraception used worldwide. There are no hormones in this device. The copper creates a sterile inflammation inside the uterus that generates a hostile environment for the egg and sperm to get together. This inflammation can cause heavier menstrual bleeding and stronger cramps than you are used to, but your menstrual cycles generally remain regular (roughly once per month).

Mirena uses progesterone to thin the lining of the uterus and thicken the mucus in both the tubes and cervix. The egg and sperm can't connect because of the thicker mucus. The thin lining means lighter periods, and many women stop having monthly menstrual bleeding with this IUD. Some women do experience irregular spotting or bleeding with Mirena instead of regular monthly bleeding. Many women, including female gynecologists, use this method of contraception for its convenience and for the benefit of having lighter or no monthly bleeding. When Mirena is removed, your periods return to normal and you can become pregnant immediately.

Some women with IUDs report that their sexual partners can feel the strings during intercourse. This is okay; the IUD is not falling out. If it is ruining your sex life, the strings can be trimmed extremely short so he can't feel them, but it might make removing the IUD more challenging later on. It is okay to use tampons while you have an IUD in place. Occasionally, IUDs fall out or move position within the uterus, but they *rarely* puncture the uterine wall, damage the uterus, or create infection. In 12 years of clinical practice, I have yet to see an IUD erode through someone's uterine wall or damage the uterus in any way.

The bottom line is that this method of contraception is a great option for many women, and fears prompted by your grandmother's horror stories should not prevent you from considering one. Talk with your doctor to see if an IUD is appropriate for you.

Before having an IUD placed, one last question to ask yourself is "How do I feel about a piece of plastic sitting in my uterus for five to ten years?" Many women understand the benefits and feel it is a great idea in theory; however, they are totally freaked out about the idea of a piece of plastic sitting inside their uterus. Every time they feel a twinge of anything (heartburn after a spicy meal, gas pains, menstrual cramps, bladder discomfort, constipation, acne, rash, hair falling out, headache, breast pain, etc.) they are absolutely convinced that their symptoms must be caused by their IUD even if the IUD has nothing to do with it. If this sounds like you, don't get an IUD. For this to be a successful form of pregnancy prevention, you must be able to have the IUD placed and then be willing to forget about it.

50.

Urban Legend

Everyone knows birth control pills make you gain weight, right? I'm sure you or someone you know gained 50 pounds while on the pill! What woman in her right mind would use pills for contraception with that awful side effect?

Weight gain is one of the most common reasons women cite for not wanting to use birth control pills as contraception. Although it is true that some women gain weight while taking birth control pills, it is also true that some women lose weight on the pill and that *most* women stay the same. Weight gain is *not* an automatic consequence of taking birth control pills. If you personally have experienced weight gain while taking pills, then this might not be an ideal strategy for contraception. If, however, you have never tried taking birth control pills and your only reason for not wanting to take them is a fear of weight gain, rest assured, this is actually extremely unlikely. Also, taking birth control pills actually *lowers* your risk of ovarian cancer!

Now for the "out of my system" myth: If you have taken pills for months or years and want to plan a pregnancy, the pill is out of your system within *24 hours*. Some women stop taking their birth control pills six months before they intend to conceive and are then shocked to find themselves pregnant five weeks later. The medication in the pill lasts 24 hours – this is why you have to take it every day for the pill to be effective. Twenty four hours after you take your last dose, there is no exogenous (outside) hormone in your body and you can become pregnant immediately!

51.

Pap Smears are Not Done in the Emergency Room

Many people falsely assume that if their pap test is normal then all of their female organs are disease free. A pap smear is a screening test for cervical cancer only. A speculum (sterilized metal or plastic disposable tube) is placed inside the vagina so the doctor can see the cervix. Then, a small brush is used to collect cells from the cervical os (opening). These cells are sent to a laboratory and examined under a microscope. If the cells appear abnormal, you will be advised to have a procedure called colposcopy in your doctor's office or a follow-up pap smear sooner than the typical screening interval of one year.

A pap smear is *not* a test for sexually transmitted infections. It is also not a test for yeast or bacteria. Don't assume you are being tested for yeast, bacteria, chlamydia, gonorrhea, syphilis, hepatitis, HIV, trichomonas, warts, HPV, herpes, or any other infection when you have your pap smear. Also, a pap smear does *not* test for uterine cancer, ovarian cancer, skin cancer, or any other female cancer. It is a test for cervical cancer only.

Additionally, a speculum exam is not a pap smear. If a speculum is placed in the vagina, it is used to look at the cervix and vaginal tissue. If this is being done at your annual checkup, a pap smear will likely be collected. If you are in the emergency room, urgent care, or doctor's office reporting a symptom such as pain, bleeding, or discharge, a speculum exam may be done, but a pap smear will not. A speculum exam in this setting is used to collect swabs to test for infection or to see where bleeding might be coming from. Many women report that they had their pap smears done in the emergency room, but this is almost never accurate.

Finally, a pelvic exam is used to check the size and shape of the ovaries and the uterus. One hand is placed on your lower belly, and one or two fingers are placed inside the vagina. The hand on the belly is used to push the ovaries and uterus down toward the vaginal hand so their size and shape can be felt. A normal ovary is sized somewhere between a walnut and a golf ball, and a normal uterus is about the size of a closed fist. Remember, a pelvic exam does not tell you if you have cancer or ovarian cysts. It can only assess whether the uterus and/or ovaries are larger than expected.

52.

Your Boyfriend Doesn't Know He Has HPV

HPV (human papilloma virus) is the virus known to cause cervical cancer. You contract this virus during sex, and it lives in the cervix and vaginal tissues. Some types of HPV cause genital warts and some types cause abnormal pap smears and cervical cancer if left untreated. Many women often discover they have HPV when they are told that their annual pap smear is abnormal. When I mention that the abnormality is from HPV and is sexually transmitted, many women immediately want to kill their boyfriends for giving them an STD. Yes, he probably did give you an STD—a dangerous one that could kill you if you develop cervical cancer—but unless he has had visible genital warts on his penis in the past, he has no idea he carries this virus.

Most men have not had warts. They carry around potentially lethal strains of high-risk HPV, give it to their sexual partners, and have no idea what they are doing. If you confront them, they deny everything because they usually haven't had any symptoms. Additionally, it can take several months for an HPV infection to cause changes in the cervix. By the time an abnormal pap is detected, the relationship has sometimes since ended. It is my experience that accusations are never good when dealing with HPV because it is nearly impossible to tell how long he or you have had the virus. My advice is to simply do the recommended treatment and follow-up advised by your doctor. Remember to get your pap smear every year and skip the conversation that starts with "You bastard, you gave me…" Now, if you are married, have no other sexual partners yourself, and suddenly turn up with chlamydia—different story!

53.

There Are Screening Tests for Only Four types of Cancer

We live in a time of many medical advances; however, despite our technology, there are screening tests for only four types of cancer: breast, cervical, prostate, and colon. A screening test means that you have no symptoms (you feel fine) and you are being screened for a given condition. One example of this is having your cholesterol tested. Having your blood drawn and tested for cholesterol levels is a screening test for high cholesterol—you feel fine but want to know if you have high cholesterol. For cancer, we have only four tests that do this: mammogram for breast cancer, pap smear for cervical cancer, colonoscopy for colon cancer, and blood PSA for prostate cancer. Notice that most cancers are not on this list. We do not have standard screening tests for lung cancer, brain cancer, liver cancer, pancreatic cancer, bone cancer, uterine cancer, ovarian cancer, stomach cancer, or the rest. For these conditions, we can only test for the condition once you present to the doctor with symptoms.

For example, if you come in saying, "I am having trouble breathing," and you are coughing up blood, an X-ray or chest CT scan will be ordered based on your symptoms of trouble breathing and coughing up blood. If a tumor is seen on the imaging, a diagnostic test such as a biopsy can then be done to find out if you have lung cancer. However, we do not have a screening test for lung cancer. We don't do yearly X-rays on everyone who has lungs to see if they have lung cancer.

In the gynecology office, I am often asked by patients to order a screening test for ovarian cancer. Although there are many ideas under investigation, we currently do not have a standard screening test for ovarian cancer. If you have certain symptoms, we could check the size, shape, and characteristics of your ovary with ultrasound. If those ultrasound pictures show a mass or a tumor, we could surgically remove your ovary and then tell you if you do or do not have ovarian cancer by looking at your ovary under a microscope in a lab. Without specific symptoms, however, taking random pictures of your ovary is not recommended. We also cannot tell if you have ovarian cancer by testing your blood or examining your ovaries in the office.

What about CA125? This is a blood test most commonly used to assess whether a treatment (such as chemotherapy) is working to treat a patient who already has a known diagnosis of ovarian cancer. It is also sometimes used to detect recurrence of ovarian cancer in women who were previously diagnosed. It is not useful as a screening test in women who have no symptoms or who have never been diagnosed with ovarian cancer. Having watched many lovely women die of this disease after a late-stage diagnosis, I hope in my lifetime to see a good screening test for ovarian cancer implemented into the standard of care. Unfortunately, for now, there is no such thing.

54.

What's up There, Mom?

If you are having a procedure or a pap smear, I recommend that you not bring children to the appointment. Often, the nurse cannot look after them, and the moment you put your feet in the stirrups, the baby starts screaming and the kids run wild. As soon as they know you are incapacitated, they cut loose! Some kids open the exam room door while you are naked on the table. Some go directly for the biohazard waste container full of used speculums and other (sometimes bloody) instruments. Some peer over my shoulder and ask, "What's up there, Mom?" And some empty all the items out of your purse and out of my exam table drawers.

We are obstetricians. We love kids. It is, however, a bit of a challenge for us to keep you modest and for you to keep control of your children during a gynecologic exam. Maybe once a year, I observe kids sitting quietly in chairs behind a curtain while Mom has her exam, but this is not the norm. Sometimes the office staff can help, but don't assume the nurse can provide child care while you are compromised.

If you do bring your children, chances are they will be looking over my shoulder with curiosity. This leads to questions you may not want to answer later, and also to imitation. This means that you may find your child suddenly trying to look up your skirt or up the skirts of girls on the playground because they saw me looking under the drape in the office. This is natural if it happens; however, it can lead to crying children on the playground and some unusual parent-teacher conferences. If you see your child imitating a gynecologic exam, please do not yell or punish, but remind your child that this is only for adults in the doctor's office.

55.

Understanding Your Pap Smear

Abnormal pap smears are very common. Colposcopy with biopsy to assess abnormal pap smears is very common (I usually do at least one colposcopy every day in my office). Even removing abnormal cells with a "LEEP" or "Cone" procedure is common. Cervical cancer is rare. Many people come to their annual exam and report a history of cervical cancer. They state, "I had cells removed from my cervix for cancer," and truly believe they had cervical cancer when, in fact, they had dysplasia (abnormal cells that are *not* cancer).

It is true that, if left untreated, dysplastic cells can become cancer; however, most women with cervical cancer have had a special type of hysterectomy (radical hysterectomy) done by a specialized surgeon (gynecologic oncologist) and are not having routine pap smears in the general gynecology office. It hurts me to see so much confusion regarding pap smear results. It seems that either people believe they have a diagnosis of cancer when they really had dysplasia (abnormal cells that are *not* cancer), or they feel they had nothing to worry about and left their high-grade dysplasia untreated, putting themselves at real risk for cervical cancer.

Be sure you understand exactly what your pap and/or biopsy results mean and what the recommended treatment options are for your given condition. It is totally reasonable to schedule a special appointment or to ask questions before or during your procedure to be sure you clearly understand your exact diagnosis. Below is a basic description of pap smear results and what they mean. If your pap smears have always been normal you can skip to the next section. If not, please read on…

A pap smear is a screening test for cervical cancer. The results can be reported as normal, atypical, low grade, high grade, or cancer. If you get a normal result, you will be advised to have your next pap smear in one to three years, depending on your age and medical history. If you have a cancer result, you will be referred to a specialized surgeon called a gynecologic oncologist for treatment. If you get a result of atypical, low-grade, or high-grade cells, you will be advised to have colposcopy (a microscope test) in your doctor's office (not in an operating room).

Colposcopy is a test that uses a microscope to look at your cervix in the office and to take additional tissue samples (biopsies) that are smaller than the tip of a pen. Most women do not feel these biopsies being taken. The biopsy results are then sent to a lab and reported as: normal, CIN1, CIN2, CIN3, or cancer. CIN stands for cervical intraepithelial neoplasia and is *not* the same as cancer. Sometimes women tell me they had stage 2 cervical cancer when what they really had was CIN2 (not cancer).

A normal or CIN1 biopsy result means you will most likely be advised to have a pap smear again in six months. A CIN2 or CIN3 biopsy result means you will most likely be advised to have a procedure (usually a LEEP or Cone procedure) to remove the abnormal cells so they do not become cancer. A cancer biopsy result means you will be advised to meet with a gynecologic oncologist for additional treatment. Following a LEEP or a Cone procedure, you will generally be advised to have a follow-up pap smear in three to six months. Clearly abnormal pap smear results can be intimidating and confusing; talk openly with your doctor and be sure you understand exactly what the results mean for your health.

56.

Your Hysterectomy: Was it Really Total?

Many women have hysterectomies (surgical removal of the uterus) for various reasons. This was more common in the past several decades than it is now, thanks to minimally invasive treatment options for abnormal uterine bleeding. A hysterectomy can be done abdominally (through an open belly incision), vaginally (through your vagina without opening your belly), laparoscopically (using cameras and instruments through small poke holes in your belly), or robotically (using a surgical robot through an incision in your belly).

A total hysterectomy among *physicians* means your uterus and cervix were removed and you still have your ovaries. A total hysterectomy among *nonmedical* people often means the ovaries were removed too. When a nonmedical patient tells a physician she had a total hysterectomy, the physician will often ask, "Do you have your ovaries?" We are not being smug or not listening. We know you just told us you had a total hysterectomy, but in our lingo, "total" means a different thing.

Doctors consider that there are four types of hysterectomies:

1. A total hysterectomy, which means the uterus and cervix, but *not* the ovaries, were removed.

2. A supracervical hysterectomy, which means the uterus was removed but the cervix and ovaries are still there.

3. A radical hysterectomy, done only by a specialized surgeon called a gynecologic oncologist, to treat cervical cancer. This type of hysterectomy involves removal of

the lymph nodes, tissue around the cervix, and a portion of the upper vagina.

4.   Any type of hysterectomy with a BSO, or bilateral salpingo-oopherectomy, which means that the tubes and ovaries were also removed. You can have a total hysterectomy with/without BSO, a supracervical hysterectomy with/without BSO, or a radical hysterectomy with/without BSO.

Many patients ask, "Can't you tell on the exam if I have ovaries or not?" The answer is, sometimes yes. Ovaries can be easily felt in women who are extremely thin and not yet in menopause. If you are of average body size and/or in menopause, the ovaries are much more difficult to feel, as they typically shrink after age 50–55. Often, the ability to distinctly feel an ovary in a postmenopausal woman implies that the ovary is larger than it should be and that further assessment may be advised.

If you have had a hysterectomy and are not sure whether you still have ovaries or not, contact the surgeon who did the procedure and ask for a copy of your operative note. If the surgeon is no longer in practice, the hospital where it was done should have a copy of the operative note on file. If you don't want to bother tracking this information down, sign a records release with your current provider and ask them to obtain the operative note on your behalf.

57.

If You Want to Be Seen on Time

If you want to be seen on time, book the first appointment of the day. Doctors are notoriously late for appointments and rarely run on time in clinic. This is because we never know what concerns or issues you have in advance or how long they will take to address during the appointment. When asked if they have any questions or concerns to discuss, some women state they have none while others pull out a notebook or typed document in 10 point font listing numerous issues.

Quite frankly, we have a difficult time cutting people off mid-sentence or mid-procedure to stay on schedule. This is especially true for gynecologists who work in a specialty that requires them to be on call for patients admitted to the hospital, emergency surgery, or labor. We could easily be rushing out of the office mid-pap smear to deliver a baby. For all providers, and especially on-call providers, if you want to be seen on time, book the first appointment of the day. We often do not have time to get behind schedule if you are first.

Likewise, if you want extra time with your doctor, request it. Most offices have set amounts of time for appointments. For example, in my office, if you come in for your annual exam and pap, you are scheduled for 30 minutes; if you are there to be checked for a yeast infection, 15 minutes. These are set in advance so that the nonmedical people who answer the phone and schedule appointments know what to do.

If you have a long list of things you would like to discuss, or if you know that you will need additional time with the doctor, simply ask when you schedule your appointment. Ask the receptionist how much time you have been allotted for your appointment. If you think it is not enough, request more. As providers, we do not want to be rushed any more than you do. We want to thoroughly address your concerns and answer all your questions. If you do not request extra time and have a long list of issues, we will often ask you to return for a different appointment to address all your concerns instead of running too far over our set time and subsequently disrupting all the down-line appointments.

58.

Don't Wait Until Your Insurance Is Ending

Believe it or not, many women come in on the 25th of the month, stating that their insurance is ending on the 30th and they need to schedule a major surgery immediately. They are then infuriated when this cannot be arranged. Any person who is interested in surgery must first have a consult to describe their symptoms and have a thorough evaluation. In the case of hysterectomy, this evaluation might include an ultrasound (often done at a later date), blood tests (often drawn in a different facility), a pap smear (results not available for a week), and an endometrial biopsy or sampling of the uterine lining (results not available for 7–10 days). Once this information is collected, a follow-up appointment is arranged to discuss the results and review the relevant treatment options. The treatment options might include hysterectomy, but a different, less invasive strategy might be advised first. In fact, some insurance plans require that other treatments be tried and fail before they will approve payment for major surgery.

Once the decision for surgery is made, there are consent forms, insurance forms, and health forms to review in detail. If you have chronic conditions such as diabetes or high blood pressure, you may be asked to see your internist and to get medical clearance for surgery prior to the operation. This means we must make sure it is safe to operate on you. Finally, major surgery requires two surgeons—your doctor and an assistant—and must be planned on a surgery schedule. Typically, a gynecologist operates one or two days per week.

From the time your workup is complete to the time you actually have surgery could be 2–6 weeks, depending on how often your specific doctor operates and when his or her assistant is available. Clearly, these things take time. It can sometimes be 3–6 months from the time of the initial consultation to the time of the operation if your insurance has specific requirements. Often, things happen faster, but I encourage you not to wait until the last minute to come in for an evaluation. Your doctor cannot and should not scramble around to operate on you on short notice unless you require emergency surgery. Painful periods may seem like an emergency to you; however, chances are they have been going on for several months or years and will require a comprehensive workup prior to major surgery. If you truly are bleeding to death from your menstrual periods, you might need emergency surgery; however, this situation is thankfully extremely rare.

59.

Don't Assume That Your Doctor Does the Procedure That You Want

Obstetrics and gynecology is a very broad field, and each doctor often has a certain area of expertise or a set group of procedures that he or she specializes in. For example, I specialize in pregnancy, office gynecology, weight loss, and I have a special interest in cosmetic procedures including Botox and Juviderm injections. One of my partners does gynecology only (no obstetrics) and specializes in gynecologic surgery. I perform NovaSure (a treatment for abnormal menstrual bleeding) in the operating room but not in the office. I have not been trained to place Implanon or how to perform Essure (a procedure that places small coils in the fallopian tubes and is a newer method of having your "tubes tied") whereas several of my office partners do these procedures. I do not do any incontinence evaluations in the office or incontinence procedures in the operating room. One of my partners specializes in infertility. She, however, does not do any incontinence evaluations. On the other hand, another one of my partners specializes in incontinence and also does cosmetic injections. Each of us has our own area of expertise, yet we all work in the same office.

When you call to make an appointment for a given problem (let's say you are having difficulty becoming pregnant), even if you have seen me in the past for an annual exam and pap smear, my partner who specializes in infertility is going to be your best option. Avoid blindly making an appointment with a doctor you have seen in the past without asking the scheduler if it is something that doctor can help you with. If you have incontinence, ask for an appointment with the office provider who specializes in incontinence, even if it is not someone you have seen before. This will save you both time and money, as you will be evaluated by the correct person from the start. Likewise, if you are interested in a specific procedure, say Essure or Implanon, ask for an appointment with the person in the office who does these procedures most often.

60.

Call Ahead

Babies don't make appointments; they come out whenever they want. This could be 3 a.m., when I am sleeping; 7:30 a.m., when I should be walking my dogs; noon, during my lunch meeting; or 2:30 p.m., during your office appointment. If your doctor delivers babies, understand that your appointment may get rescheduled or postponed. I know this is a hassle, especially if you have been waiting three months for your pap smear, but there is no great solution. Obstetrics is an unpredictable business. Certainly, days that your doctor is "on call" for labor and delivery are more likely to be delayed, so scheduling your appointment for a non-call day is one idea.

The easiest way to take charge of this situation is to simply call the office a few hours before your appointment and ask how things are going. Ask the receptionist if your doctor is running on time or if he or she has anyone currently in labor. If you know there is someone in labor, then you have the option to reschedule and/or to be prepared to wait longer than expected for your appointment. If it seems there is likely to be a delay, ask the scheduler if you can arrive at a later time so you don't have to wait, keeping in mind that women push anywhere from three minutes to three hours during childbirth. As obstetricians, we understand that our schedules are inconvenient for you (they are for us, too), and we don't intentionally want you to wait. You can be proactive in helping us be respectful of your time by calling ahead, especially if you know the provider you are scheduled to see is on call.

Similarly, your doctor may be tired and working less efficiently on his or her post call day (the day after he or she has potentially been up all night). If you want a well-rested provider, consider *not* scheduling your appointment—or especially your surgical procedure—on your doctor's post call day. Oddly enough, airline pilots have required rest times, as do truck drivers; however, physicians and surgeons do not. I can get up at 5 a.m., see patients in clinic all day, stay up all night with women in labor, and then appear at 9 a.m. for your major surgery with no sleep, no questions asked!

My advice, therefore, is for you to request a date for your surgery when your surgeon has not been on call the night before. This will give you a better chance at a rested physician. Of course, you can't avoid fatigue at all costs (your doctor might have been up all night with his or her own sick child, or awake because her spouse was snoring…who knows). At least you can eliminate one variable if you take out the on-call factor. I don't know how many of the alleged millions of medical errors reported each year could be avoided if doctors had the same rest requirements that pilots do, but my guess is that fatigue leads to many unnecessary mistakes, and being proactive about scheduling surgery can help you protect yourself.

61.

If You Report Something Abnormal, We Will Advise Further Testing

Many women come in and describe a complaint that warrants further evaluation. For example, every woman over 40 who reports irregular periods, heavier bleeding than usual, or bleeding lasting 12 days will generally be advised to have additional testing. This may include an ultrasound, a sampling of the uterine lining (endometrial biopsy), a gynecologic exam, a pap smear, and/or blood tests. It will then be up to her whether to proceed with the recommended evaluation. Your doctor often cannot tell you if what you have described is normal without further testing.

Many patients state, "I don't want any tests; I just want to know if this is normal." I'm not trying to run up your medical bills, but it is nearly impossible for me to tell you if your symptoms are related to a serious condition or not without a comprehensive workup. This is like asking your auto mechanic to tell you why the engine makes a rattling sound when you drive over 40 miles per hour without letting the mechanic look under the hood or drive the vehicle to hear the sound. The purpose of any given test is to figure out if what you have described is normal or not. For example, heavy, irregular menstrual bleeding could be normal or could be cancer. It could also be any number of easily treated benign conditions such as thyroid disease or polyps; however, I can't be sure of the diagnosis without doing an evaluation.

The same goes for many other complaints, including breast pain, belly pain, pain with sex, and vaginal discharge. I can rarely tell from your description alone if you have a yeast infection, an allergic reaction to panty liners, or chlamydia. An exam, at least, is warranted, and most likely a swab to assess for yeast, bacteria, trichomonas, chlamydia, and the like. I can guess what's causing your symptoms, but I would rather do a proper evaluation and advise an appropriate treatment. Your best bet is to prepare for a medical exam at every appointment.

62.

Line up a Chauffeur for Office Procedures

Once, following a procedure, I observed a patient falling on her way out of the office, hitting her head on a table, and requiring stitches in the ER. Don't let this happen to you! If you are having an office procedure, it's best to have someone else drive you to your appointment. Most office procedures are easy, quick, and uncomplicated; however, just as some people pass out while having their blood drawn, a similar reaction can occur during a gynecologic procedure. If you are prone to this, if you took Valium prior to your appointment, or if you are extremely anxious about the procedure, have someone drive you. The last thing we want is for you to crash your car over an office procedure or to pass out in the waiting room.

When an IUD is placed, for example, the inside of the uterus is touched with a plastic tube; this can give a sensation of cramps, nausea, or dizziness for some, and nothing of notice for others. If you are injected with numbing medication prior to a biopsy, that can cause shaky legs, rapid heartbeat, and lightheadedness. Any procedure such as office hysteroscopy (looking inside the uterus with a camera), Essure (a type of permanent sterilization), or NovaSure (a treatment for abnormal uterine bleeding) in which you receive narcotic pain medication or sedation prior to the appointment also requires a chauffeur.

Frequently, people come in for a given procedure, drive themselves, and then feel they are going to return to work immediately. For some, this is no problem; however, it's best not to assume this will be the case for you. You may not be able to

return to work for several hours, so don't schedule your procedure 30 minutes prior to an important meeting or an annual
performance review with your boss. The smartest strategy is to
have someone drive you, to advise your employer that you may
not be back, and then see how you feel. We are happy to provide
a note to be excused from work or school for the day, following
most procedures.

63.

RN: The Office Bouncer

Every physician has a nurse or medical assistant who usually does far more work than the physician to keep the office running smoothly and is the primary patient liaison. Typical responsibilities of the nurse are to prepare exam rooms, assist with office procedures, answer patient phone calls, refill medications, report abnormal lab results to the physician, and notify patients of their results. This means that if you come into the office for a chlamydia test or a cervical biopsy, the office nurse is the person who will most likely call you with your results. Nurses are trained to do this and work closely with physicians. My office nurse is invaluable, and I could not imagine trying to run a medical office without her.

Sometimes doctors receive complaints such as, "Some nurse called me about test results; I thought the doctor would do that," or "Since when does the doctor not call his or her own patients back?" Keep in mind that it is standard practice for the office nurse to field patient phone calls and to answer medical questions herself. Similarly, it is standard practice for the nurse to send letters or to call patients with their test results.

If you hear from an office nurse, this does not mean the doctor feels you are not important or is ignoring you in any way. If I answered every patient phone call myself (sometimes 20 or more per day) and called back every test result individually, I would be on the phone all day and would not be able to evaluate patients in the office. Remember that the nurse is not the office bouncer or the physician's bodyguard. One of her primary clinical responsibilities is to speak directly with patients about their concerns and test results. She can often help triage over the phone whether you need an appointment or have a situation that can be handled otherwise.

64.

Your Medical Record Belongs to You

You have a right to read your medical record. It cannot be kept secret from you. If you wish to read your medical record or have a copy, simply ask the front office staff to help you. Sometimes there will be a minimal charge for processing. Similar to your credit report, reviewing your medical record periodically is a good idea so you can make corrections, ask questions, and see what type of information is being provided to insurance companies. This is critically important when it comes to so-called preexisting conditions.

For example, let's say you were medically treated for headaches but never had a formal diagnosis of migraine or other specific type of headache. The word "headache" is a symptom and does not pin you down to a diagnosis that could be considered a preexisting condition limiting future insurance. In contrast, if you had one or two appointments for headache and a diagnosis of "complex migraine headache" was made, now you have a diagnosis and possible preexisting condition.

As physicians, we primarily use the medical record to document our interactions with patients for future reference, as patients are often uncertain about exactly what procedures they had or exactly what medications they took. We use it as a tool to communicate with other physicians and insurance companies. It is not secret information about you (as implied in the *Seinfeld* episode), and you are welcome to a copy at any time.

If and when you read through your medical record, be sure to ask your doctor to explain terms or diagnoses that you don't understand. I once spoke with a very angry woman over the words "smoking cessation" written in her chart. She was upset that I had labeled her as a smoker after she had worked so diligently to quit. In reviewing the medical record with her, I explained that the words "smoking cessation" in the context of what I had written actually meant that she had quit smoking. If you read something confusing in your record, ask the doctor for an explanation, as many medical terms can be misinterpreted.

65.

Insurance Fraud

Did you know it is insurance fraud to comp a friend or family member for a medical appointment? This means that if you are my best friend, cousin, or coworker and I see you for a medical appointment in my office, I have to write a chart note and charge you the exact amount I would charge a complete stranger for the same service. If I write a note and don't charge you or if I charge less than I would charge a stranger, I am committing insurance fraud and can go to jail for this. *Jail!* Really.

The only way to comp someone for a visit is to not document any portion of the visit, as if it never existed. This is never a good idea. For one, there is usually a record of your appointment through the office schedule. Additionally, what if you have a complication related to the condition or treatment I prescribed and there is no record of your evaluation? If you see a doctor who is a friend or family member, don't expect him or her not to charge you for the visit. We love you, we want to help you, but we really don't want to go to jail.

Similarly, we cannot generally write prescriptions for people we have not officially evaluated for a given condition and docu-mented an assessment in a medical chart. This means that you should not call your neighbor, Dr. Smith, and ask him to pre-scribe Diflucan for your suspected yeast infection on Saturday because you don't want to wait until Monday for a medical appointment. Unless he comes to your house, evaluates you for yeast, and writes a note in your medical chart, he really shouldn't prescribe a medication for you. If you are an established patient of Dr. Smith (have seen him or one of his partners in the office before as a patient) and he is the on-call doctor, then that is a different scenario and he can most likely prescribe Diflucan. He should not also fill your husband's asthma inhaler or little Jimmy's ear drops because you are going out of town. This type of prescribing behavior is frowned upon by credentialing entities and is not safe medical practice. Be respectful of your physician friends and family members and don't ask them for random prescriptions because it is easier than having a standard evaluation.

66.

No News Is Not Good News

I once cared for a patient who had advanced cervical cancer on a pap smear and unfortunately died within a year of my diagnosis. When I asked what her result was from the year prior, she stated that she had never heard anything from the doctor so she assumed her pap result was normal. I went back and reviewed the records from the prior physician and discovered that indeed her prior pap had never been reported and the only one on record was normal from more than three years prior. This entire problem (and cancer diagnosis) might have been avoided if the patient had been diligent about receiving her results when the lab or doctor dropped the ball. Yes, receiving, reviewing, and reporting results is absolutely our obligation, but you can help yourself and your doctor greatly by making a follow-up phone call if two weeks have passed from your appointment and you haven't heard anything. Computers are computers, and humans are human. Medicine is a world of computers and humans and even at our best important information still gets misplaced at times.

The bottom line is that if you have an ultrasound, blood draw, mammogram, pap smear, biopsy, or any other medical test, be absolutely sure you receive and understand your results. People often assume that no news is good news when, more often, no news means that the result slipped through the cracks. All offices try to keep track of results and to explain them in a timely manner; however, inevitably, some are overlooked or lost or never get reported from the lab. Being proactive about receiving results can ease your mind and who knows, it just might save your life!

67.

How to Use the Doctor on Call

All ob/gyn medical offices should have a doctor on call. This means the doctor carries a phone or a pager to answer emergent questions and to help you decide if you need to go into the emergency room after hours. The best reason to use the on-call physician is if you have a serious problem (for example, heavy unexpected bleeding, severe pain, inability to urinate, something stuck in your vagina). The on-call doctor can advise you whether to go to the ER immediately, to try a certain strategy at home, or to arrange an office appointment in one to two days. The on-call physician can help you avoid spending hours in the emergency room for things that can be relieved at home or in the office. Likewise, he or she can advise immediate treatment in the ER and help you get evaluated urgently if indicated.

If you ran out of birth control pills, think you have a yeast infection, or can't feel your IUD strings, these are best assessed in the office and do not require a phone call to the doctor at 3 a.m. Of course, you can always call any time with any concern and we will happily help you if possible. Keep in mind that many issues cannot be resolved over the phone and that when you call, we will often advise you to make an appointment or to go to the emergency room. I often have women call with belly pain or vaginal irritation and want me to tell them over the phone why it is occurring. Other times, women call and want to know if their IUDs are in the right place. A diagnosis for these and other similar symptoms requires a physical exam and cannot be made over the phone; an appointment will likely be advised.

If you do contact the on-call physician after hours, keep in mind that it may be through an answering service or paging system.

This means that a nonmedical person or a computer system will be taking your initial call. Simply tell that person your name, phone number, and doctor's name. You do not need to describe every detail of your vaginal bleeding to the operator or answering service. They usually do not pass that information along to the on-call doctor. When I receive a page after hours, it states a phone number and sometimes a name, with no other information. If you have just explained your entire problem to the operator, you may feel frustrated that you have to re-explain it to me. Also remember to answer the phone when we call back. Oddly enough, I receive many urgent pages that I cannot return because no one answers the call, the voicemail box is full, or the phone number provided is incorrect or not in service.

68.

Come in Immediately

If you are advised to come in to the office or hospital immediately, please do so. It amazes me how many people call with seemingly serious complaints such as difficulty breathing, heavy bleeding soaking their clothes, or severe abdominal pain and then don't want to come in for evaluation. I will receive a call stating, "I am in severe pain and can't stand up." I will advise the person to come in to the emergency room or office right away and will get a response such as, "I can't leave work right now," or "I don't have transportation." I'm never sure how to interpret these comments. Does this mean that I need to send an ambulance to your job site, that you are really not in pain because you are continuing to work, or that your boss is so outrageous that he or she is forcing you to work despite your critical condition?

Often, people want a diagnosis and solution over the phone without an evaluation. This is possible in certain situations, but serious symptoms such as trouble breathing or severe pain require immediate attention. How do I know through the phone that you are not developing a blood clot in your lung or rupturing your appendix?

The same applies to trips scheduled out of town. If you call your doctor and report that you are experiencing something serious (severe abdominal pain, heavy bleeding, difficulty breathing) and we advise you to come in for an evaluation immediately, this generally means that you should not get on an airplane instead of driving to the hospital. Often women call and report something seemingly serious and then become angry when we advise evaluation. Further discussion usually reveals that coming in to the hospital means missing an important date, a trip out of town, or a work event. Doctors are not intentionally trying to ruin your plans, but it is often impossible to complete a proper assessment (especially of something potentially serious) over the phone. I have had women ignore advice for immediate evaluation, get on a plane, and end up in a hospital out of town during their vacation. Don't let this happen to you!

69.

The Dreaded Disability Forms

Give your provider plenty of time to complete paperwork or disability forms. Much to my dismay, paperwork is part of medicine. In fact, I often spend more time charting, dictating, writing letters, signing forms, and completing paperwork than I do actually delivering babies, operating, or seeing office patients. I expect that there will be a given amount of paperwork to complete for every patient I see. This includes disability forms, proof of pregnancy letters, insurance forms, physical papers for school or work, adoption papers, and more. Often, these papers can be completed while you are in the office for your appointment; however, do not assume this is the case. Allow your provider at least one or two days to complete your requested paperwork. Many of the forms take 30–60 minutes to complete properly and cannot be done the same day without asking all the patients scheduled after you to wait an additional 30–60 minutes. If you need to pick up certain documents at the time of your appointment, call ahead and let your provider know, or drop them off a few days in advance so the proper scheduling arrangements can be made.

Afterword

My intention in writing this book was to inform and entertain all the women in the world who have ever visited or will visit a gynecology office. As a women's health physician, I spend much of my time encouraging, evaluating, and treating women with various conditions. Often, I find myself marveling at how much misinformation is carried around as seemingly common knowledge despite its inaccuracy. After years of shaking my head, I finally sat down and wrote this book to help you understand your own body, to dispel common myths, and to help you get the most out of your gynecology office appointments. I appreciate comments or feedback sent to info@RedLetterHealth.com so I can make subsequent editions more informative, comprehensive, and understandable.

In addition to my western medical obstetrics and gynecology practice and specialty weight management clinic, I speak professionally throughout the year, and also work with phone clients as a holistic health coach on the issues of fatigue, low libido, depressed mood, insomnia, and stress management. If you would like to inquire about health coaching or book a speaking engagement, please visit www.RedLetterHealth.com or call 406-219-3537.

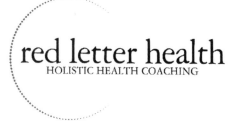